Gender and Sexuality in Ireland

Gender and Sexuality in Ireland

John Gibney (ed.)

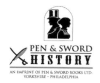

PEN & SWORD
HISTORY

AN IMPRINT OF PEN & SWORD BOOKS LTD.
YORKSHIRE – PHILADELPHIA

First published in Great Britain in 2019 by
Pen & Sword History
An imprint of
Pen & Sword Books Ltd
Yorkshire - Philadelphia

Hardback ISBN: 9781526736796
Paperback ISBN: 9781526769558

A CIP catalogue record for this book is available from the British Library.

Typeset in Ehrhardt MT 11/13.6 By SRJ Info Jnana System Pvt Ltd.

Printed and bound in the UK by TJ International Ltd.

Pen & Sword Books Ltd incorporates the Imprints of Pen & Sword Books
Archaeology, Atlas, Aviation, Battleground, Discovery, Family History,
History, Maritime, Military, Naval, Politics, Railways, Select, Transport, True
Crime, Fiction, Frontline Books, Leo Cooper, Praetorian Press, Seaforth
Publishing, Wharncliffe and White Owl.

For a complete list of Pen & Sword titles please contact

PEN & SWORD BOOKS LIMITED
47 Church Street, Barnsley, South Yorkshire, S70 2AS, England
E-mail: enquiries@pen-and-sword.co.uk
Website: www.pen-and-sword.co.uk

or

PEN AND SWORD BOOKS
1950 Lawrence Rd, Havertown, PA 19083, USA
E-mail: Uspen-and-sword@casematepublishers.com
Website: www.penandswordbooks.com

Contents

Preface

The history of sexuality in Ireland remains relatively understudied when compared with the more well-worn paths of political and military history, but that is not to say that it has never been studied. Now, in the fourth instalment of the 'Irish perspectives' collaboration between Pen and Sword and *History Ireland*, a range of experts explore Irish history from the perspective of the broad concept of sexuality, in both theory and practice. From the legalities that defined gender roles in the middle ages and early modern periods, to women's role in political life and civil society, concepts of patriarchy, population change, the role of prostitution in Irish life, incarceration, infanticide, abortion, homophobia, attempts to impose - and ignore - Catholic morality in independent Ireland, struggles for women's rights and reproductive rights, the culture wars of the 1980s, and Irish people simply trying to have good sex lives, the essays gathered here cast light on aspects of Ireland's past that are often neglected in more mainstream narratives of Irish history.

The chapters below have all been drawn from the archives of *History Ireland*, and re-edited; with regards to illustrations, every effort has been made to contact rights holders. If we have missed any, the error will be rectified in any subsequent edition.

Contributors

Art Cosgrove was formerly president of University College Dublin.

Mary Cullen formerly lectured in history at Maynooth University.

Geraldine Curtin completed her Ph.D at NUI Galway on juvenile crime and poverty in Connacht in the nineteenth century.

John Cunningham lectures in history at NUI Galway.

Diarmaid Ferriter is Professor of Modern Irish History at UCD.

John Gibney is a historian with the Royal Irish Academy's Documents on Irish Foreign Policy series.

Paul Gray formerly lectured in history at Queen's University, Belfast.

Mary Kenny is an author and journalist.

Liam Kennedy is emeritus professor of history at Queen's University, Belfast.

Angus Mitchell lectures in the Kemmy Business School at the University of Limerick.

Mary Muldowney is a founding member of the Oral History Network of Ireland and is Historian in Residence with Dublin City Council.

Mary O'Dowd is Professor of Gender History at Queen's University, Belfast.

Clare O'Halloran lectures in history at University College Cork.

The late Margaret Ó hÓgartaigh lectured in history at All Hallows College, Dublin.

Clíona Rattigan completed her Ph.D at Trinity College Dublin on single mothers and infanticide in twentieth century Ireland.

Paul Ryan lectures in sociology at Maynooth University.

Brendan Scott is editor of *Breifne: Journal of the Breifne Historical Society.*

Jim Smyth lectures in sociology at Queen 's University, Belfast.

Introduction

John Gibney

In 1966, on the Irish broadcaster RTÉ's iconic *Late Late Show*, a newly married Irish woman admitted on live TV to not wearing a nightdress on her honeymoon. This prompted a good deal of public fulmination, most famously the declaration by one parliamentarian, Oliver J. Flanagan, that sex had only come to Ireland since RTÉ, the state TV station, had been established. Often misquoted as 'no sex in Ireland before the *Late Late Show*', the furore can be taken as symbolising a particular form of attitudes towards sexuality in independent Ireland.

Of course, if Flanagan had been right, there would hardly have been an Irish public to be offended. There can be no human history without sexuality, though there has been plenty of history written without it. Yet it can be difficult to use sexuality as a category of inquiry in history without clarifying how it is to be used. Does it mean sexual and/or gender identity, in a subjective sense? Or the way gender roles can be objectively defined by social norms, not to mention the law? Does it relate to the basic reality of human reproduction? Sexual pleasure? Or the policing of sexuality by authorities of various kinds? All of the above can be grouped under the loose term of 'sexuality', and all of them are explored to some degree in the chapters that follow.

The history of sexuality in Ireland remains understudied, and often overlaps with the history of gender. This can sometimes be taken as shorthand for 'women's history'; a category that serves as a necessary corrective to histories of Ireland that have silently excluded the lives and experience of women, as explored in Mary Cullen's opening chapter. The bulk of the remaining essays deal with the period after the 1801 Act of Union, but Art Cosgrove and Brendan Scott explore the manner in which gender roles and sexuality were corralled within the legal requirements of marriage and divorce in the medieval and early modern periods, and which shaped the degree of political, economic and social influence that women could wield. In the eighteenth century women were excluded from formal political power, yet as Mary O'Dowd reveals, women remained politically committed and active in less formal, but no less meaningful, ways.

Contrasting studies of the roles played by women in nineteenth and early twentieth century Ireland follow, in the form of their exclusion from civil society in the form of the Royal Irish Academy (explored by Clare O'Halloran), and

Maria Luddy's overview of prostitution in Irish society. The most basic function of sexuality – reproduction – is examined by Peter Gray and Liam Kennedy in their study of population change in County Clare after the Great Famine. Many of the themes they highlight (illegitimacy and 'illicit sexuality') are also touched on in Geraldine Curtin's study of the policing and institutionalising of gender in Victorian reformatories.

These chapters deal with one form of sexuality. Two pieces by Angus Mitchell, from 1997 and 2016 respectively, address another: the ongoing controversy over the sexuality of the former colonial administrator and republican Roger Casement, who was executed in August 1916 for conspiring with the Germans prior to the Easter Rising of that year. The fact that diaries detailing a range of homosexual encounters were used to blacken Casement's reputation and thus derail appeals for clemency prior to his execution remains one of the most contested issues pertaining to sexual identity in Irish history. The awkward possibility of accommodating a gay patriot was a step too far in the conservative society of post-independence Ireland, which helped to foster the assumption that the diaries must have been forged. Equally, this could be seen as nothing to be ashamed of, and Casement has assumed the status of gay icon. The question of their authenticity remains unresolved – Mitchell's perspective is simply one side of the argument and has been contested vigorously by the veteran Northern Ireland LGBT activist Jeffrey Dudgeon and others – though the traditional conflation of Casement's sexuality with their veracity is not automatically a given. Given the legal restrictions on homosexuality that pertained for so long in Ireland (under British rule and otherwise), the controversy over Casement offers a rare opportunity to highlight an otherwise hidden strand of Irish life.

Discussions of sexuality in independent Ireland often focus on the imposition of Catholic morality in the Irish Free State and its successor republic; and that is no myth. The Catholic Church in Ireland was preoccupied by sexual morality. As shown in Jim Smyth's chapter on controversies over dancehalls and that of Margaret Ó hÓgartaigh on the alleged moral danger of womens athletics, the boundaries of public morality were policed vigorously in a society that slowly but surely restricted the participation of women in public life (a fact that was not lost on many Irish women). More tragic realities are revealed by Cliona Rattigan's accounts of both infanticide and unofficial abortion in independent Ireland.

There then follow chapters by Diarmaid Ferriter and Paul Ryan that pose a challenge to the assumption that a stultifying Catholic morality was accepted unquestioningly. The correspondence with the agony aunt Angela Macnamara reveals a world in which Irish people were actually trying to have good sex, and presumably, some were succeeding.

The final chapters by Mary Kenny, John Cunningham and Mary Muldowney deal with the challenges faced in the 1970s by the movements for women's rights, and reproductive rights (neither of which can be divorced from the other). The recent referenda that legalised same-sex marraige in 2015 and which removed the constitutional ban on abortion in 2018 could be seen as marking a liberalisisation in attitudes to sexuality and reproductive rights. It is fitting, in the wake of the 2018 referendum, that this anthology ends with Muldowney's oral history of the bitterly divisive 1983 campaign that introduced the now-defunct eighth amendment granting equal legal status to the lives of mother and unborn child.

There are, of course, gaps in this the overview provided here. In relation to gender roles, there is little on the role of women in philanthrophic organisations, or even in artistic and cultural life. There is nothing on the works of authors such as Edna O'Brien. Nor do the campaigns for women's rights of the early twentieth century that became intertwined with the upheavals of the Irish revolution feature (though these have attracted attention in the course of the ongoing 'Decade of Centenaries'). The chapters here also tend to deal with the twenty-six counties that gained independence in 1922; and the Catholic conservatism found south of the Irish border that had much in common with what existed in Northern Ireland. The 'architecture of containment' that survived in independent Ireland - 'Mother and Baby' homes, 'Magdelene Laundries', and 'industrial schools', administered by the Catholic Church (and occasionally its Protestant counterparts) with the connivance of the state - and the appalling sexual abuse revealed within this network in recent decades does not feature here. Nor, Casement notwithstanding, do LGBT identities and experiences. Yet this is not to dwell on shortcomings; rather, it is to highlight how much else there is to study under the broad rubric of 'sexuality' in Irish history (and recent initiatives such as UCD's 'Industrial Memories' project, exploring the industrial school network, and the pioneering Irish Queer Archive, are welcome developments). The study of Irish sexuality remains relatively understudied, but what the following articles hopefully reveal are some of the realities that can be uncovered by exploring Irish history from the perspective of this most fundamental aspect of humanity.

Chapter One

'History women and history men': The politics of women's history

Mary Cullen

T he development of women's history grew directly from the contemporary feminist movement. The roots of feminism lie in the behaviour-patterns societies have prescribed for women and men. While these have differed over time and place, feminism has always grown from women's perception that the sex roles prescribed by their own society conflicted with their knowledge of themselves and with their development as autonomous persons.

The new wave of feminism which emerged in Western society around 1960 challenged the prevailing stereotype which insisted that every female, by virtue of her sex, was individually fulfilled and made her best contribution to society solely as a wife and mother, subordinating the development of other talents and leaving responsibility for the organisation of society to males. The American Betty Friedan called this model the 'feminine mystique', and women around the globe recognised it as corresponding to what they knew in their own cultures.

Feminist rejection of the feminine mystique was challenged by the assertion that history showed that women had always been satisfied with this role. Since history books seldom mentioned women at all, with the exception of a few monarchs and revolutionaries whose lives and careers hardly conformed to the mystique model, feminists turned to the historical evidence with the question: what did women do? The answers which have come so far, and they are only the beginning, raise wide-ranging challenges to establishment history.

As feminist enquiry focuses on different areas of knowledge, history included, the first stage is seeing and saying that women are invisible in the knowledge and theory of the particular discipline. Next comes the search for 'great' women, individuals who have 'achieved' within the criteria by which men are judged to have 'achieved'. From this the focus moves to the contribution of a wider range of women to political, social and intellectual movements which underlie patterns of continuity and change in societies. The fourth stage sees women as a group, defined by their shared female sex, demanding the attention

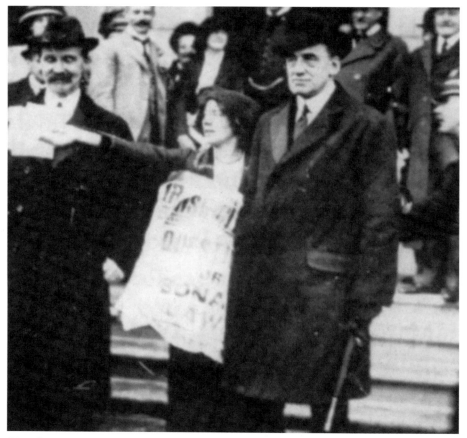

Meg Connery of the Irish Women's Franchise League attempts to hand suffragist leaflets to Andrew Bonar Law (left) and Edward Carson (right).

of historians. This development has a radical potential to which this essay will return. The ultimate stage should be the writing of a new integrated history incorporating the historical experience of both sexes.

Let us consider the implications of one early discovery by feminist historians: the women's emancipation movements of the nineteenth and early twentieth centuries and the causes that gave rise to them. While feminist movements were neither the central nor the most important phenomena in women's history, their existence allows us to bypass one regularly repeated explanation for the invisibility of women in so many history books. Since women were not participants in public politics, historians, it was asserted, could hardly be blamed for not dealing with them. The women's emancipation movement, a highly visible and international political movement, refutes this explanation.

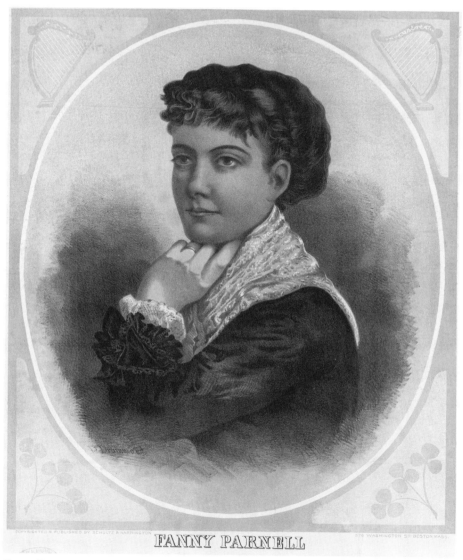

Fanny Parnell: Irish poet, Irish nationalist, and the sister of Charles Stewart Parnell.

While laws, regulations and customs were not identical in all countries the position of women relative to men was fundamentally similar. In virtually every country in western society, women were excluded from political life, whether by holding public office, or as members of parliaments, or as voters. They were barred from higher education and the professions. Titles and property passed to sons in preference to daughters. The home was seen as 'the woman's sphere',

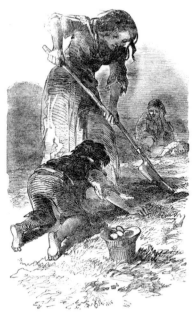

Irish women at work in the fields in nineteenth-century Ireland. (Illustrated London News)

yet, to take a representative example, under English common law, in force in Ireland, when a woman married her legal identity merged into that of her husband. Her property, whether earned or inherited, passed under his control to dispose of as he pleased and the law gave him full authority over her and their children. Divorce was considerably more difficult for a wife to obtain than it was for a husband, and if a woman left her husband his duty to maintain her lapsed while his right to her property did not. In sex-related offences such as adultery, prostitution and illegitimate birth, the law treated women as the more guilty and punishable party.

In campaigns starting around the middle of the nineteenth century and continuing into the 1920s and 1930s, in country after country, feminists revolutionised the status of women by removing most of the legally imposed civil and political disabilities based on sex. By any standards it was a sizeable achievement even if with hindsight we know that the underlying stereotypes of 'natural' or 'correct' feminine and masculine behaviour were harder to shift.

One aspect of this rediscovered history of the women's emancipation movement is its relevance to women's self-knowledge today; its restoration of part of their lost 'group' memory. It tells us that we have not been paranoid in perceiving oppression, and that the problem of sexism has older and deeper roots than many have realised. On the more positive side, the better sexism

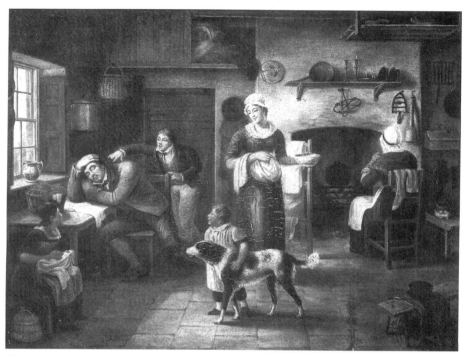

The family as a woman's workplace: 'A kitchen interior', by John Mulvany.

is understood, the better the chance of eliminating it. Further, the history of the women's emancipation movement establishes beyond doubt that relations between the sexes, including relations of power, have not been unchanging throughout history and dispels the belief that women have always conformed happily to a 'natural' role of passivity and subordination. It places current feminism in context as part of a long historical process, rather than the historical aberration often suggested. Feminists today can start from the knowledge that women before them dissented from imposed patterns of behaviour and changed them. It frees them to build on what is already there instead of re-inventing the wheel in each new generation.

It also raises the question of why all this had to be rediscovered in the first place. Why had it ever been lost? Why has the historical reality that the structures of Irish society included a systematic limitation of women's autonomy and freedom of action, a limitation not applied to men, gone unrecorded in histories of Irish society? It is difficult to see why an organisation of society which gave men a monopoly of access to political and economic power, and excluded women from virtually every avenue of approach to these, should be something that historians have not seen as a significant or important aspect of Irish society.

It is equally difficult to see how feminist organisation to abolish sweeping civil and political disabilities could be regarded as more sectional, more trivial or less significant than, for example, nationalism or the labour movement.

It appears that the answers are not to be found in the content of the historical record but in the minds of historians. If we dismiss a conspiracy theory of deliberate suppression, the explanation can only be that most historians have not seen women as important or 'significant' in the history of their societies. They have written history within a paradigm that sees men as the active agents in the patterns of continuity and change historians look for. This paradigm does not see women as an integral part of human society, but as peripheral and essentially outside history. Once the question 'what did women do?' was seriously asked, it became clear that this paradigm blinkered historians' vision and distorted findings and interpretations.

Women's history and feminist studies in general continually remind us that knowledge is not an objective given but a human creation. Historians do not exist in a vacuum but are members of a society, formed by it and influenced by its value systems. If they bring with them ways of looking at the world which see males as 'doers' and 'leaders' and females as 'passive' and 'followers' they are unlikely to look for evidence of action or change brought about by female initiative, and may fail to recognise its significance when found.

This raises the question of bias in the writing of history. History written from the perspective of groups distant from centres of power and privilege, such as women's history, labour history, Marxist history, black history, is often labelled as 'political' and liable to bias. The pitfalls of bias are real. As a feminist historian I am likely to want to find certain things, and there is always the temptation to search more assiduously for the evidence that supports one's hypothesis than for that which refutes it. But knowing my bias puts me in a better position to be alert to this danger and to try to avoid it. Others too will be more alert to see and tell me if I fail. But historians who believe themselves to be value-free and 'neutral' are in more danger. An assumption that the current political or intellectual status-quo or orthodoxy is usually 'right' and those who dissent from it likely to be 'wrong' is as political a perspective as a feminist or Marxist one and, if unconsciously held, more likely to distort the way history is written. In my own case I am more concerned about the biases and value-systems I inevitably have, but of which I am not aware, than I am of feminist sympathies.

The realisation that women as a group have a history displaying patterns of continuity and change grew from the mounting evidence that differences in the relative position of men and women in societies could not all be attributed simply to 'nature' or 'biology' This can be illustrated by two examples from nineteenth-century Irish history — at one end of the social spectrum the landed family of the Parnell's in County Wicklow in the second half of the century, and at the other end widowhood and illegitimate birth in the 1830s. The brother and sisters Charles, Fanny and Anna Parnell were all committed and active nationalists. Charles went to a public school and to the University of Cambridge, inherited an estate, entered parliament and became the leader of a political party. All these stages in his life were open to him as a male. As females his sisters could not go to a public school, go to Cambridge, enter parliament or become leaders of political parties. The circumstances of Anna's leadership of the Ladies Land League vividly illustrate these differences. Fanny and Anna did not inherit estates but had incomes settled on them by their father and charged on the estate of another brother. These contrasts in the political, social and economic consequences of sex were not determined by 'biological' difference but by the laws, regulations and customs which determined what males and females could and could not do at that place and time in history.

At the other end of the social scale the Poor Inquiry of the 1830s found among the categories of the destitute two which contained no men, but only women and children. These were widows with families of young children and illegitimate children and their mothers. Again, no direct biological imperative decreed that among the poorer classes widows, but not widowers, with young children, and illegitimate children and their mothers, but not their fathers, were highly likely to be destitute. Here also the causes must be sought in the distribution of resources at that time and place, in who controlled that distribution and in whose interests, and within terms of what paradigm of society, class structure and male–female relationships.

With the revelation that there have been real political, social and economic differences consequent on being born a male or a female at a particular time or place, and that these differences have varied from one society or culture to another and changed over time, sex emerged as a category of historical analysis. This was not sex in the sense of biological determinism but in the way societies create sex roles to which individuals are socialised or coerced to conform. The word 'gender' was drawn into use to denote the social construction of sex.

Used with precision within specific historical contexts, gender is a valuable concept in historical research and interpretation. It focuses attention on the relationships between the sexes, how these are structured and maintained and how they change over time and place. It also directs attention to relationships within the sexes, those between different groups of women and between different groups of men. It enables the historian to apply the concept of sex as a social construction in research and interpretation. Historical specificity also makes it clear that gender does not stand on its own as the only important analysis. It interacts with other factors such as class, colour, nationality, ethnic origin, political affiliation, religion, age, marital and parental situation and many more, in locating individuals or groups in their historical context. Feminist historians argue that, while gender is not the only essential analysis, it is one of the essential analyses, and that, if it is excluded, the picture drawn by the historian will be to a greater or lesser extent distorted.

Thus defined and used, gender analysis forestalls reductionist interpretations that all women have shared the same history, or that women's history is simply a history of the oppression of all women by all men. Women have been oppressors both as individuals and as members of oppressing classes or nations. Men have been oppressed, by other men and by women, as well as being oppressors. Women's history is far more than oppression and resistance to it, important as both these aspects are.

The German historian Gisela Bock explains how feminist historians have challenged 'three dichotomies in traditional thought on gender relations', those of nature versus culture, work versus family, and public versus private. The nature versus culture dichotomy sees men and male activities as 'culture' and a proper subject of historical study, but sees women and female activities, especially those connected with sexuality, women's bodies, pregnancy and motherhood, as 'nature', unchanging over time and place, and so outside the historian's remit. Feminist research has challenged this by showing that the words 'nature' and 'culture' have not had fixed immutable meanings but have meant different things at different times and places and are in reality interrelated and interdependent.

The second dichotomy sees family life not as 'work' but 'natural'. But families were and are work places for most women, where they bear and raise children and care for family members. The bread-winner husband who supports his family is himself supported by his wife's work. This switches attention to the more real dichotomy of the inequalities in the valuation and reward of women's work and men's work.

Nor does the third dichotomy of public versus private withstand scrutiny. Men cannot operate as they have traditionally done in the public world without the support of the private world. As Bock points out, 'male workers, male politicians and male scholars perform their tasks only because they are born, reared and cared for by women's labour'. Instead of men and women occupying separate worlds which proceed in parallel, there is only one world where the political, economic and social are interdependent, and where gender relations interact with all three.

This brings to the forefront the question lurking in the background so far, the question of men in history. History as it has been written has been less the history of men than the history of the activities of privileged groups of men who occupied positions of public power. It has seldom looked at men as a group, the subset of humanity defined by their male sex. Just as the history of women cannot be written without reference to gender relationships, neither can the history of men.

Women's history has made it untenable to see the male role in society as the human norm, from which women were for some reason, whether 'biological' inferiority, slower cultural development or whatever, left behind in human evolution and so had to try to catch up with me. The interdependence of the gender roles of the sexes rule out this interpretation. The re-evaluations to which this will lead are ongoing. One will certainly focus attention on definitions of what is recognised as significant historical change and the respective contribution to it by individuals or groups in positions of public power and by individuals and groups far distant from such locations.

They are also likely to include re-assessment of the contribution of the full-time male politicians, intellectuals, artists, soldiers, revolutionaries or whatever who have been all these full-time because of women's work. Male privilege, control of resources and freedom from daily family responsibility undermine theories which incorporate the idea of the 'naturalness' of male 'achievement' and which cite in support the relative paucity of similar female achievement.

Instead of asking why women have dissented, it might be more useful in increasing our understanding of the past to ask why male elites have so consistently tried to keep control of wealth, education and political power as male monopolies, and to limit women's freedom of action by expanding their childbearing capacity into a life-time career devoted exclusively to care of family and home at the expense of any serious participation in the affairs of society at large or sustained commitment to intellectual or artistic endeavour. Can the pronouncements by so many of the 'great masters' of western philosophy on the intellectual and moral inferiority of women as compared to men continue to be dismissed as unimportant hiccups which do not affect the overall evaluation of their systems of thought? By whose instigation and in whose interests did the dualities and theories of opposites that have bedevilled western thought about the sexes come into being? Why has male identity so often been built on being different to and having control over women? What impact have male sex-role stereotypes which see aggression and dominance as acceptable or desirable masculine characteristics had on the history of different societies?

This leads on to the big question of how a more embracingly 'human' history will be written. Seeing relationships between the sexes as an integral part of the history of a society will be central. We can also hope that women's history will carry into all areas of research and interpretation its concern with the origin and operation of systems of power and control, as well as its openness to the complexities of human experience and to the danger of imposing absolutes and dichotomies, not only when dealing with women and men but throughout the search for the past.

Who then is going to write the new integrated history and when? One view is that first we need to build a sufficient base of publication in women's history to provide a firm foundation. Then, once a critical mass of knowledge and theory has been reached the patriarchal paradigm at present in possession will collapse under the weight of the increasing mass of contrary evidence, and leave the way open for a new paradigm within which historians can rewrite history.

Some developments in recent decades suggest that vigilance may be needed to prevent the radical potential of women's history being diverted into a *cul de sac*. These include a tendency to misuse 'gender' as a synonym for 'women', a misuse which allows the essence of gender analysis, that sex is a social construct, to be bypassed and allows men as a group to again elude the historian's scrutiny. This can produce a descriptive social history, valuable in the information it gives, but which does not ask the 'hows' and 'whys' which push social, economic and political history into engagement with each other.

Particularly ironic is the emergence in the United States of 'gender history' as a rival to 'women's history', complete with claims to be more universal and less biased. Since women's history led to the concept of gender history, it is hardly surprising that the sceptical see this new dichotomy as an attempt to neutralise the challenge of women's history by marginalising it as less than fully academically respectable.

Here I believe the politics of women's history come into play. Today's women's history, including the concept of gender, came from today's feminism, a movement which asserts women's autonomy and responsibility and challenges male and female sex-role stereotypes which limit these and which incorporate male dominance over women. The diversionary movements described above appear either to fail to understand the concept of sex as a social construct, or to fail to engage with it, and may be seen as elements of a counter-revolution.

It is arguable that historians who do not understand current feminism will have difficulty in accepting that women's history is 'real' history, and so a real part of human history, however well-intentioned they may believe themselves to be. It may be going too far to suggest that women's history and an integrated human history can only be successfully written by feminists, whether they be women or men. However, I am convinced that, if the potential of women's history is to be realised, the historians concerned need to at least understand feminism today, whether or not they agree with its analysis. Unfortunately it appears that most historians, like most people generally, see feminism as essentially women wanting to be like men, and so as a 'women's issue' which need not involve men. Believing this is an effective defence against having to think about feminism seriously, and in particular about its challenge to men and male stereotypes.

If my argument has any validity, it follows that, in tandem with the work of research and publication, we need a debate about the nature of women's history and its methodologies and politics. The objective will be to put this debate on the agenda of historians of women and from there to move it on to the agenda of the wider community of historians.

Chapter Two

Marriage in medieval Ireland

Art Cosgrove

Medieval Ireland was, according to contemporaries, a country divided into two 'nations'. On the one hand there were the descendants of the Anglo-Norman settlers of the late twelfth and early thirteenth century, on the other the successors to the older Gaelic Irish population. The church reflected this division and was split into two sections, one *inter Anglicos* (among the Anglo-Irish), the other *inter Hibernicos* (among the Gaelic Irish). We must therefore investigate marital behaviour in the two parts of Ireland, the section of the country under English law, and the Gaelic Irish area where the old brehon law still held sway.

Church law on marriage was defined and clarified during the twelfth and early thirteenth centuries. Basic Christian teaching was straightforward – what God has united, man must not divide (Mark 10:10). But how do you know when God has united a man and a woman in matrimony, or, in other words, what constitutes a marriage? The matrimonial bond was created by the consent of the two parties, freely given, preferably expressed in a public ceremony. One of the consistent aims of the church was to have marriages publicly celebrated. But many marriages did not conform to this ideal. A public ceremony was not required to make a marriage valid and indissoluble. Because the consent of the couple rather than the church ceremony was the essential element, the church recognised unions which took place without its knowledge or blessing. The 'private' celebration of marriage had obvious disadvantages, particularly if the partners subsequently disagreed. A public ceremony safeguarded the contract. Yet because many people believed that they could regulate their marriages for themselves, clandestine unions remained common and, inevitably, produced more disputes than those which observed all the formalities laid down by the church. The church also defined those impediments which prevented individuals from validly contracting marriage. Obviously if one partner had married before and the spouse was still living, it was impossible to enter upon a second marriage. Those who had taken solemn religious vows or major holy orders were also prohibited from matrimony,

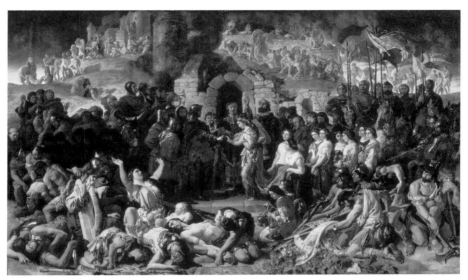

'The marraige of Strongbow and Aoife', by Daniel Maclise. (National Gallery of Ireland)

and the parties to a marriage had to have reached the age of puberty (fourteen for boys, twelve for girls) before they could make a binding contract. The church also forbade marriage between those who were considered to be too closely related. The regulations on marriage were designed for universal application throughout the western church. And since it was the church that determined what constituted or did not constitute a marriage, it was accepted that marriage disputes should he heard only in church courts. How were the regulations observed in Ireland between the thirteenth and sixteenth centuries? The evidence is not very satisfactory. The records of ecclesiastical courts do not survive for any Irish diocese, therefore we are forced to rely on the incomplete and haphazard records of marriage litigation which appear among the registers of the medieval archbishops of Armagh. From the late fourteenth to the early sixteenth century we are provided merely with glimpses of an Irish ecclesiastical court dealing with marriage disputes. This in itself means that the evidence is biased, but it is unfortunately true that marital harmony tends to leave little trace in the records.

Within Gaelic Ireland marriage behaviour had long been the target of criticism. Throughout the eleventh and twelfth centuries church reformers attacked a pattern of marital behaviour based not on the canon law of the church but on much older traditions. Thus, Irish law on marriage permitted a man to keep a number of concubines, allowed divorce at will followed by the remarriage of either partner, and took no account of canonical prohibitions regarding

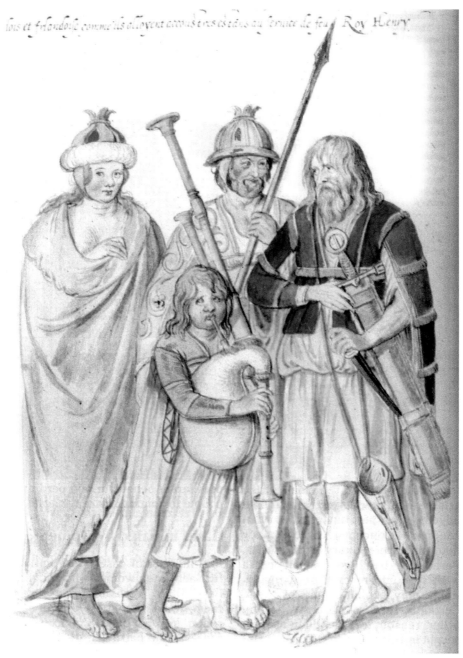

A watercolour depicting Irish attire by Lucas de Heere, c. 1547 (Central Bibliotheeek, Rijksuniversiteit, Ghent)

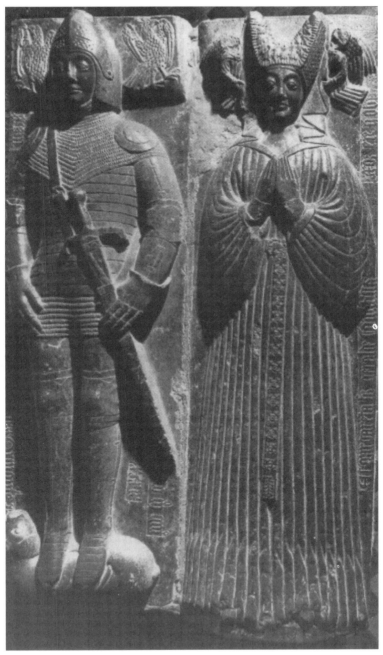

Tomb effigies of Margaret Fotgerlas and Piers Butler (eighth Earl of Ormonde) in St Canice's Cathedral, Kilkenny.

consanguinity or affinity. It is not surprising to find, therefore, that one of the benefits which Pope Alexander III hoped might accrue from Henry II's visit to Ireland in 1171-72 was a reformation In Irish marriage customs. But traditional marriage behaviour seems to have survived the coming of the Anglo-Normans, at least among the higher ranks of Gaelic Irish society. Many men and women among the aristocracy continued to have a succession of spouses and this was a key factor in the proliferation of some of the major families. For example, Pilib Mág Uidhir, lord of Fermanagh (d. 1395), had twenty sons by eight mothers and Toirdhealbach Ó Domhnaill, lord of Tir Conaill had eighteen sons by ten different women. This marriage pattern may have been confined to the upper reaches of Gaelic Irish society; lack of evidence prevents any estimate of marital behaviour lower down the social scale. For the Gaelic Irish aristocracy real difficulties were caused by canonical regulations on consanguinity and affinity. In a letter to the pope in July 1469 seeking a dispensation from impediments of consanguinity to permit Énri Ó Néill to marry Johanna MacMahon, Archbishop Bole of Armagh made the general point that several of the leading men in Ireland 'are living in incestuous relationships, because they can rarely find their equals in nobility, with whom they can fittingly contract marriage, outside the degrees of consanguinity and affinity'.

The impact of the church regulations on affinity and consanguinity was naturally much greater in small scale societies like those in Gaelic Ireland, and the frequency with which dispensations were sought is an indication of their effect. But, equally, the desire to be dispensed, often at considerable trouble and expense, shows that there were many who were not prepared to flout the church law. What was it that prompted couples to seek these dispensations? In the Anglo-Irish area the desire to safeguard inheritance rights could well have been a factor, but this was less important for the Gaelic Irish aristocracy, among whom acknowledgement of paternity rather than canonical concepts of legitimacy determined hereditary entitlements. Perhaps a troubled conscience, or a wish to conform to church regulations, may explain some of them. Certainly there can hardly be any other reason for the dispensation sought in 1448 by Aedh Ó Conchobair, described as a nobleman of the diocese of Kildare. Prior to his marriage to Honora Nic Ghiolla Phadraig he had sexual relations with both her sister and another woman related to her in the third degree of affinity, thus invalidating the union. But these affairs were unknown to Honora's friends and to all others, and the bishop of Kildare was therefore authorised to absolve Aedh, dispense from the impediments created by his pre-marital behaviour and permit the couple to contract marriage again.

A number of cases were initiated by Gaelic Irish women who sought to have their husbands restored to them, sometimes after years of separation. In

1397, Una O'Connor sought redress. She had been dismissed by her husband, Manus Ó Catháin, without any court judgement and replaced by a concubine. Katherine O'Doherty complained that her husband, Manus McGilligan, ignored the decision of the Derry diocesan court that she was his legitimate wife and openly consorted with other women. The attitude of Gaelic Irish men of rank towards the canon law and the ecclesiastical courts is best illustrated, perhaps, by the case involving Muircheartach Ruadh Ó Néill, head of the Ó Néill's of Clandeboye (1444-68). Ó Néill had married Margaret, daughter of Maghnus Mac Mathghamhna and had subsequently deserted her for a woman named Rose White. In justification he claimed that his marriage to Margaret was invalid by a tie of affinity since he had previously had sexual relations with Margaret's first cousin Maeve. In support of his contention, he brought forward the explicit evidence of one Aine 'new Owhityll', a fifty year-old woman. In her deposition she stated that Muircheartach had been captured and detained by Maeve's father, Ruaidhri Mac Mathghamhna; during the period of captivity he often had Maeve with him in bed. The witness claimed that she herself had shared the same bed, that she had often seen the couple naked together and that she was certain that sexual intercourse had taken place between them. She admitted that Maeve had not become pregnant, that she was uncertain about the date of the alleged incidents but that they had taken place within Ruaidhri's dwelling without his knowledge. But the court refused to accept this evidence, clearly taking the view that the story had been fabricated to provide a pretext whereby Muircheartach could escape from an unwelcome marriage. And although the case dragged on for over two years, the eventual decision of the archbishop of Armagh in December 1451 was that the marriage between Muircheartach and Margaret was valid; Ó Néill was ordered, under pain of excommunication, to separate from Rose White and to accept Margaret as his legitimate wife. Muircheartach was acting in a manner sanctioned by Gaelic Irish tradition. Yet clearly he felt that the canonical regulations could not be ignored; otherwise he would hardly have gone to the trouble of mounting his ultimately unsuccessful defence. Nevertheless, the clash between two quite different concepts of marriage and its function in society continued throughout the middle ages. The problem was that women regarded as concubines by the church often enjoyed the same legal and social status as wives in Gaelic society, and the children of such women were accorded the same rights as those of the canonically recognised wife.

Within Anglo-Ireland the secular legal system presented no such challenge to the canon law. Church influence was clearly greater. For instance, in the late fifteenth century when it became known that Patrick Goldsmith was living adulterously with Belle Barry in Dublin, the mayor expelled Belle from the city for a year. The measure had only a limited effect since Patrick would secretly bring Belle from Kilmainham to his room at night, but it is indicative of a desire on the part of the municipal authorities to support church rulings. The Dublin administration did attempt to regulate marriage practices in one way. Concern about the threats to the security and cultural identity of the colonial settlement posed by intermarriage with those hostile to it led to restrictions on the choice of marriage partner. The ordinance of 1351 forbade marriage between the colonists and any enemies of the king, whether Gaelic or Anglo-Irish. Fifteen years later the Statutes of Kilkenny imposed a ban based solely on ethnic grounds, prohibiting any 'alliance by marriage ... concubinage, or by caif (*coibche*)' between the Anglo-Irish and the Gaelic Irish.

Though lacking the competence to adjudicate on the validity of marriage, the secular courts did have to deal with offences that arose out of marital strife. The most notable case of this type was heard at Cork in May 1307. It concerned John Don, a wine merchant from Youghal, who married a woman called Basilia and shortly afterwards went abroad on business. During his absence Stephen O'Regan came to John's house 'asking Basilia that he might be her friend. She lightly consenting, they lay together ... for the whole time that John was abroad'. On his return John was informed by his neighbours about what had been going on and, naturally irate, he forbade Stephen to visit his house in future.

Subsequently, however, when John was absent on a business trip to Cork, Stephen again came to the house and slept with Basilia. When John learnt of this second offence, he devised a plan to trap Stephen. He had, attached to his house, a tavern and the keeper of this promised him that he would let him know if Stephen came to visit Basilia again. On a day following John pretended that he was going to Cork on business but instead went to another house in Youghal. That evening, Stephen and Basilia dined together with one Stephen Ie Jeofne, who, unknown to the couple, seems to have been an ally of John. After supper Stephen O'Regan went to the tavern and drank some wine with the tavern-keeper. While they were drinking Basilia passed through the tavern to her bedroom. Stephen and the tavern-keeper followed her. Aware now of the need for discretion, Stephen and Basilia attempted to buy the silence of the tavern-keeper and Basilia's maid by offering the former the sum of five shillings and the latter a cow. Then Stephen proceeded to take off his shoes, clearly intending to spend the night with Basilia. The tavern-keeper, faithful to his prior agreement with his employer, now went to the house of Stephen Ie Jeofne where John Don was waiting with a group of armed men. Once informed of what had happened, they proceeded to John's house, hoping to catch the guilty couple together. The noise of the armed men's approach alarmed Stephen and Basilia and they extinguished their candles. Stephen then decided to attempt an escape, but in the hall of the house he ran into John Don's armed men. They threw him to the ground, bound his hands and feet, and then castrated him. Stephen succeeded in his action for assault and was awarded substantial damages of £20 against John Don and his associates. The latter avoided imprisonment by the payment of a fine of five marks (£3. 6s. 8d.). A week later John Don counterclaimed against Stephen for compensation for goods destroyed or stolen from his house and was awarded £2 by the court.

Almost all of the other evidence for marital behaviour in Anglo-Ireland comes from the Armagh registers and is mainly concerned with the southern half of the Armagh diocese which was *inter Anglicos*, mostly contained in the modern County Louth. Suits to enforce marriage contracts formed one part of the court's business; it also had to deal with pleas for annulment, a declaration that a marriage contract had been invalid from the outset. Annulments were sought on a variety of grounds. As already noted, a plea that the parties were related within the forbidden degrees of consanguinity or affinity might be made. More often the case was based on an allegation of pre-contract, that one party to a marriage contract was already validly married and thus disqualified from making a second marriage. In cases where pre-contract was alleged, the court had to establish not only the validity of the contract but also its date so as to ensure that it was made prior to the second marriage agreement. It then had to determine whether the spouse of the first union was still alive at the time of the second contract. On occasion this might involve the court in consideration of events that happened many years before. A case in 1481 turned on evidence of what had occurred thirty years previously. Thaddeus Carpenter sought the annulment of his union with Juliana Maynaghe on the grounds of a valid pre-contract between Juliana and Roger Sarsfield. A number of witnesses claimed that they had been present either at the church marriage ceremony or at the wedding-feast of Roger and Juliana in Ardee thirty years before. The couple had lived together for some time, but Roger then left and went to live in England. He was unable to persuade his wife to join him there and she then contracted marriage with Thaddeus Carpenter 'before the Earl of Worcester came to Ireland', that is, prior to 1467. Roger's sister, Jenet Sarsfield, testified that she knew that her brother was alive five years before because she had received a letter from him asking her to come to England. For good measure she added that only three years ago she had received a message from him via Milo Fleming, a merchant from Slane, requesting her to send her son to him in England.

It is worth noting that the court always upheld the earlier valid contract. This it did even if the first marriage was made clandestinely and the second in church. While consent rather than consummation made a marriage valid, it was possible, nevertheless, to secure the dissolution of the bond on the grounds of impotence. Usually the woman pleaded her desire to be a mother and the inability of her husband to fulfil that desire, and the Armagh court did award annulments on those grounds. But the court was clearly aware of the danger of fraud or collusion and would not accept a plea of impotence without some form of substantiation, a precaution clearly justified in a case brought by Anisia Gowin in February 1521. In the previous December Anisia had failed in her bid to have her marriage to Nicholas Conyll nullified on the basis of pre-contract. She now charged her husband with impotence, a charge he denied. The court ordered that she was 'to spend the night with Nicholas in the same bed, without any disturbance' and appointed nine men to carry out an inspection of Nicholas and report their findings. Their evidence left no doubt as to Nicholas's ability to perform his marital duties. Even when the man admitted impotence the court demanded corroboration from seven witnesses.

Overall the surviving records of matrimonial litigation among the Armagh registers support the view that marriage practices in Anglo-Ireland did not differ markedly from those elsewhere in Latin Christendom. In Gaelic Ireland practices did diverge significantly but the corollary was a heavy demand for the sanction of canon law. In general, despite the best efforts of the church authorities, marriage was still widely regarded as a personal matter subject to a private contract between the parties. Clandestine unions remained common; and even after the Council of Trent's decree outlawing such unions in 1563, clandestine marriage was to have a long history in Ireland.

Chapter Three

Career wives or wicked stepmothers?
Marriage and divorce in the Pale

Brendan Scott

Arranged marriage alliances were a very important feature of life in the Pale in early modern Ireland. Rather than springing from emotional attachment, marriage among the gentry and nobility was normally viewed as a contract fostering mutually beneficial alliances between the families involved. A marriage had to be advantageous to both families and was normally contracted to consolidate land holdings or to increase wealth. It was also possible, through marrying into nobility, to receive a title or to curry favour with the Crown. So choosing a suitable spouse was obviously a very important task and not one that could be undertaken lightly. The six marriages of Jenet Sarsfield, a member of a Pale merchant family, brought her further into the upper echelons of Pale society and, along the way, into confrontation with one of her stepchildren. Her marriages and those of her fourth husband, Sir Thomas Cusack, who experienced his own set of marital problems, serve as a useful template for the discussion of just what those who brokered marriage alliances wished to achieve, as well as some of the problems that they could encounter along the way. Jenet Sarsfield was probably born in the late 1520s or early 1530s, the daughter of John Sarsfield of Sarfieldstown, County Meath. One of her brothers, William, later became an alderman of Dublin. Her first marriage was to Alderman Robert Schillingford, mayor of Dublin in 1534–35, with whom she had one daughter, Katherine, her only child to reach adulthood. When Robert died, Jenet married James Luttrell, who died in 1557. She was pregnant with James's child when he made his will that year, but this child did not survive for long, if indeed it was brought to term at all. Jenet's third husband was Robert Plunkett, baron of Dunsany, from whom she received her title 'Lady' and, following his death, 'Lady Dowager'. Her marriage to Robert was short-lived, and when he died in 1559 Jenet made her fourth marriage that same year, this time to Sir Thomas Cusack of Lismullin, County Meath. Jenet's fifth and penultimate husband, John Plunkett, died in 1582, leaving Jenet to marry John Bellew, her sixth and final husband, whom she predeceased.

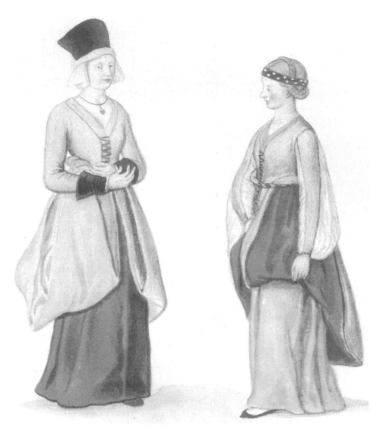

Lucas de Heere's watercolour of townswomen ('Femme et fille Irlandaises') c. 1547. (Central Bibliotheek, Rijksuniversiteit, Ghent).

Thomas Cusack had been made lord chancellor of Ireland in 1550 and was an influential political figure in the Pale. Born around 1505, Cusack was in his mid-fifties when he married Jenet, who was probably in her late twenties or early thirties at this time. Financial comfort was obviously a major consideration for people who married in the early modern period, and the marriage between Thomas and Jenet, which was childless, is a perfect example. When Cusack married Jenet, the financial implications of the match were made perfectly clear. In a feoffment dated 2 November 1564, Thomas settled lands upon her 'in consideration of the preferment that I the said Sir Thomas had with Dame Genet Sarsfield in maryadge and in consideration of dyvers great sums of money that the said Jenett laid out and paid for such debts as I did owe to the Queenes majesty and others, and for dyvers other good considerations and profitable things by her extended to mine use'.

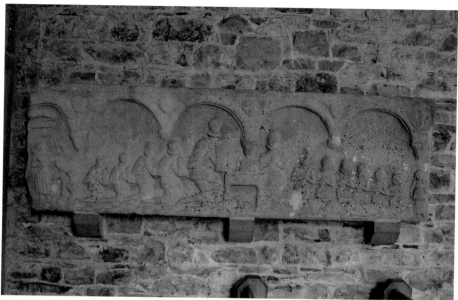

Section of Thomas Cusack's funerary monument, now in Tara Church, Co. Meath, showing Cusack, his second wife Maud Darcy, and their thirteen children. Elsewhere it has the coats of arms of the Cusack's, Darcy's and Sarsfield's (family of his third wife, Jenet) but no reference to his first wife, Joan Hussey, or her family. (Julian Thomas/OPW)

   Cusack also experienced his own share of marital woes, which he attempted to obscure as much as possible. In his will, he refers to Maud Darcy, who predeceased him, as his first wife, but this was not actually the case. His first wife was in fact Joan Hussey, with whom he had three children. Thomas later applied for a divorce from Joan on grounds of consanguinity (they were third cousins), which was granted in 1537. Interestingly, Cusack was accused in 1547 of persuading a servant of his to 'enter into familiaritie with his wif [Joan Hussey] whereupon he had a divorse betwixt him and hir: and soone upon married the late wife of the baron of Skeyne [Maud Darcy]'. This accusation, however, was part of a series of allegations designed to smear Lord Deputy Anthony St Leger and his followers, so it should not necessarily be taken at face value. Although lessened from seven degrees of blood relationship to four in 1215, the laws of consanguinity and marriage relations were still strict in the sixteenth century. If a man had had sexual relations with a woman, he could not then marry her sister, first, second or third cousin. Nor, through bonds of spiritual affinity, could a widower marry the godmother of his children or vice versa.

   Thomas and Joan were not the only couple to ignore these regulations in early modern Ireland. The Elizabethan church set forth its 'table of kindred and

The letter written by Edward Cusack to William Cecil, Elizabeth I's secretary, in 1580, outlining his stepmother Jenet's links with the major families of the Pale.

affinity' in 1563, requiring every church to carry a copy, which they often failed to do, indicating the continuing levels of confusion regarding consanguinity. Commenting in 1584, Richard Stanihurst noted that the native Irish were only then beginning to take notice of the marriage laws regarding consanguinity. As Thomas Cusack and Joan Hussey were probably always aware of their close blood relationship, it is difficult to understand why they had married in the first place. Claiming that their original marriage was invalid, however, was not an uncommon tactic utilised by estranged marriage partners who wished to remarry.

The Reformation brought some changes in marriage laws in Ireland. The Irish parliament of 1540–41 passed the 'Act for marriages', which decreed that from 1 July 1540 a solemnised and consummated marriage should supersede an unsolemnised and unconsummated prior contract. This was to safeguard against marriages agreed by oral contracts (often used by men attempting to satisfy their immediate carnal desires). The law was repealed in 1549 on the grounds that it instead encouraged people to break contracts in order to consummate their relationships.

Joan Hussey remarried after her divorce from Cusack, and, describing her as 'sometime my wife', Thomas left money for her in his will in return for goods that he had received on her behalf, possibly her dowry. The likelihood of an acrimonious split is supported by Cusack's funerary monument, which only contains the coats of arms of the Cusack, Darcy and Sarsfield families, with no reference to his union with Joan and the Hussey family. The denial and admission in his will of his first marriage also illustrates Cusack's own ambivalence regarding the failed union. This invalidated marriage continued to cause difficulties for Cusack's heirs into the 1630s, when a great-nephew of Thomas, one John Cusack, petitioned for Thomas's estates on the grounds that Thomas's children with Maud (there were thirteen) were illegitimate, as his separation from Joan had been unlawful. John even alleged that Thomas himself had destroyed the dispensation document in an attempt to hide this accusation. Although John's litigation ended in failure, it is indicative of the problems that beset the families of those affected by divorce, even 100 years after the fact!

Few marital breakdowns in Tudor Ireland, however, were as scandalous as that of Cusack's second wife, Maud Darcy. Rumours spread of Maud's involvement in the death of her first husband, James Marwarde, baron of Scryne, in September 1534. It was alleged that Maud Darcy had Marwarde murdered by Richard Fitzgerald, whom she subsequently married. Fitzgerald, however, was later attainted and executed for his role in Kildare's rebellion, after which Maud quickly married Cusack. Maud's extramarital affair was not the only one to end in bloodshed in Ireland's early modern period. Nicholas Eismonde from Wexford was pardoned in 1557 'for the manslaughter of Richard Eismonde, gent., whom he had found in criminal conversation with his wife and who was endeavouring to escape from the house by force'. These notorious cases were very much the exception, however, which merely heightened the sense of scandal when they did occur.

Despite precautions taken by Thomas to prevent such an occurrence, litigation between his children and his widow broke out after his death. To Thomas's son, Edward Cusack, Jenet Sarsfield must have seemed like the archetypical wicked stepmother. For her part, Jenet obviously viewed her string of spouses as career moves—marrying was her profession, and she did it for financial gain. It seems that there had been tension between Jenet and Edward even before Thomas died, and upon the death in 1571 of his father, Edward became embroiled in bitter legal disputes with his stepmother over the conditions of the will. Thomas had obviously envisaged trouble between both parties upon his death and stated that 'if he [Edward] objects to these arrangements he is to have none of the goods but only land to the value of 200 m.p.a.'. Jenet, on the other hand, was to benefit financially from any such protest that Edward was to make.

Nevertheless, Edward was determined to cause problems for his stepmother and claim what he saw as rightfully his. Jenet was left many of Cusack's personal effects, as well as the nunnery of Lismullin, which came into Thomas's hands in the early 1540s following the monastic dissolutions some years earlier. Edward broke into the house while Jenet was away and stole some items, along with 125 cattle. As a result of his actions, Jenet sued him in chancery, provoking Edward to retaliate in kind. Jenet further alleged that Edward 'ran away with the said will [of Thomas] and being pursued did cast the same in a field of corn'. He later retrieved the will and 'blotted it in sixteen several places' in an attempt to destroy its more contentious passages. Despite his protests to the contrary, Edward was found guilty of stealing a casket of jewels and, unable to pay the damages that he owed to his stepmother, was forced to return the jewels that he had earlier sworn he had not stolen from her. It was discovered later, however, that the jewels had been willed by Edward's mother, Maud, to her children, who had never received them, so it seems that Edward was merely retrieving what was rightfully his and had been withheld from him by Jenet.

By December 1573 Edward had obtained a chancery decree against Jenet and her new husband, John Plunkett, ordering them to hand over to him the manor of Lismullin and its profits since Thomas's death. This was not the end of litigation between the parties, however, and during 1579–80 Edward once again sued Jenet and John Plunkett. It was at this time, while in England, that Edward sent a genealogical account of Jenet's relationships with important personages in the Pale to William Cecil, secretary to Elizabeth I, in the hope of settling the dispute in his favour. This letter demonstrates quite clearly how many of the important Pale families were interrelated. If you opposed one, as Edward did, you were in danger of pitting yourself against some of the most powerful families in the Pale. Although Janet eventually vacated the manor, she allegedly ransacked it of most of its possessions, destroyed the orchards and brought with her the title-deeds that should have been left in Edward's possession. Edward then sought to retrieve the title-deeds and compensation for his losses, but his involvement in the Nugent conspiracy of the early 1580s seems to have brought his lawsuit to a halt.

Although Jenet was left most of Thomas's wealth, widows were legally only supposed to get one third of their husband's income (the 'widow's third'). The large amount bequeathed to Jenet by Thomas was therefore one of the probable reasons why Edward was so unhappy. The third due to the widow rose to half if there were no children or if the children had already been 'preferred', i.e. taken care of financially. A widow had common law right of dower for her life in a third of her husband's lands, but this right was increasingly waived in favour of a settled jointure. Not everyone was happy with the 'widow's third', however, and one John Burnell neatly sidestepped this obligation. He paid his widowed stepmother, Joan Talbot, full rent from some of his lands once every three years; this meant that for the other two years he had full access to the rent due from the property. It also meant that John only had to pay her once every three years, and not at all if she remarried or died during this three-year period, an arrangement that was highly satisfactory for John but disadvantageous for Joan. This example illustrates how some exploited loopholes in the system to their own benefit and to the detriment of some widows.

When Jenet eventually died in February 1598 she was commemorated as 'Lady Dowager', a title to which she was entitled through her marriage to Lord Dunsany and which she used throughout her life. Moreover, Jenet was buried alone, not with Robert Schillingford or Dunsany, who had given her a daughter and a title respectively; Clodagh Tait has suggested that her long career as a wife entitled her to this privilege, and her solitary interment does seem to indicate an unusual degree of autonomy.

By and large, it appears that their parents and guardians often used sons and daughters to further their family's prospects and social standing. Once made, these ties were normally strong, and rarely broken. Disputes such as those between Jenet Sarsfield and her stepson Edward, however, illustrate the difficulties facing those individuals who, through numerous tactical marriages, strove to improve their financial and social positions. As so many Pale families were connected through marriage, it was inevitable that personal rivalries and animosities could have repercussions for all the families involved. The ambiguous legal and social position held by some whose marriages ended in separation must have made them rue their wedding day, and the scandal and intrigue that went hand in hand with extramarital affairs would have put a great strain on many interfamilial relationships. Sometimes marriage caused as many problems as it was deemed to solve.

Chapter Four

Women and patriotism in eighteenth-century Ireland

Mary O'Dowd

Francis Wheatley's painting of the Irish House of Commons in 1780 is well known and has been reprinted many times. It celebrates the occasion of Henry Grattan's speech during the debate on the rights of the Irish parliament in the spring of 1780. The painting provides a striking visual record of an important political event while at the same time capturing the sense of splendour and drama of the Irish parliament during the most important decade of its existence. The painting is divided into two sections: the lower half portrays the MPs in the chamber of the Commons, while the upper half focuses on the crowded public gallery. Some of the men in the chamber and in the gallery are, like the main figure, Grattan, wearing Volunteer uniforms. A striking feature of the painting, not often commented on by historians, is the presence of women in the gallery. A close look at the women also reveals that one of them is dressed in a Volunteer uniform, while others appear to be wearing Volunteer colours in their dress or hats. Regretfully, although we have a key that identifies most of the men in the picture, no list of the women is known to exist. We cannot, therefore, identify the woman in uniform, although we can say that she appears to be wearing the uniform of a Dublin-based regiment.

The presence of the women in the parliamentary gallery is intriguing and raises interesting questions as to why they were there and what their presence at this important debate tells us about gender, politics and patriotism in eighteenth-century Ireland. Were the women in the gallery for the social occasion, viewing the proceedings in the same way as they would view a theatrical performance, or were they more actively engaged with the politics being discussed? And why is one of the women dressed in a military uniform?

One answer to the question as to why women were in the gallery or, more specifically, why the artist, Francis Wheatley, chose to depict them in the way he did is that he was paid to do so. Wheatley was an English artist who came to Ireland in the late 1770s. His arrival coincided with the beginning of the

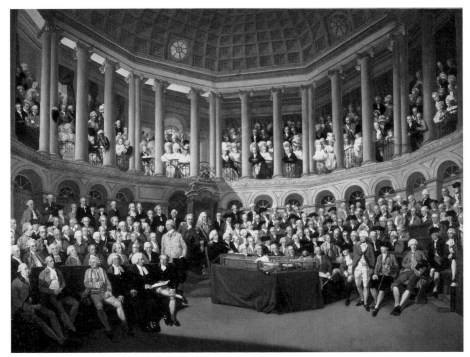

Francis Wheatley's painting of the Irish House of Commons in 1780 provides a striking visual record and captures the sense of splendour and drama of the Irish parliament during the most important decade of its existence. A striking feature of the painting is the presence of women in the gallery. One is dressed in a Volunteer uniform, while others appear to be wearing Volunteer colours in their dresses or hats. (Leeds Museum)

Volunteer campaign of the late 1770s, and Wheatley quickly recognised the commercial possibilities of the Volunteer movement for an enterprising artist. The House of Commons painting is one of several that Wheatley undertook of people and events associated with the Volunteers. In November 1779 he had completed his large painting of the duke of Leinster's review of a Volunteer regiment in front of parliament in College Green. The painting was successfully sold through public auction and purchased by the duke of Leinster, and can today be viewed in the National Gallery of Ireland. Encouraged by the sale of this picture, in the months following the 1780 constitutional debate Wheatley planned a second public painting. He advertised in Dublin newspapers his intention of composing a painting of the parliamentary debate and invited those who attended to come to his studio to sit for the painting. Wheatley charged people for the privilege of being included in the painting and planned to sell it by public auction.

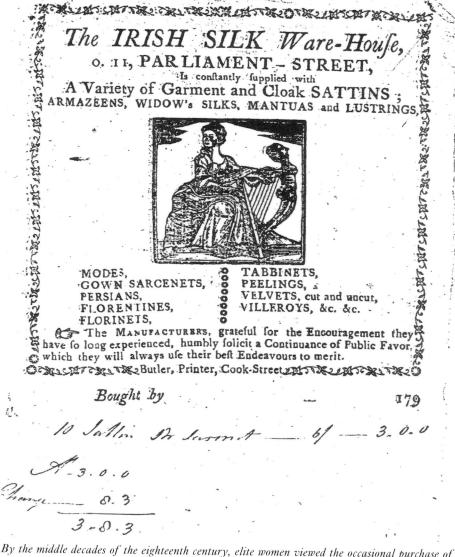

By the middle decades of the eighteenth century, elite women viewed the occasional purchase of Irish-produced textiles, such as advertised here, as an appropriate form of public charity. (Walker's Hibernian Journal, June 1779)

Wheatley's House of Commons painting was, however, never finished. Rumours circulated in Dublin that the painting had been over-subscribed and that more people wished to be included in it than the artist had room for on his canvas. It was alleged that Wheatley was painting over some of his

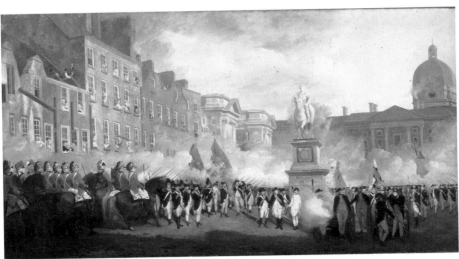

The Dublin Volunteers on College Green by Francis Wheatley. Women can be seen in the windows overlooking wearing Volunteer colours, one in a Volunteer uniform. (National Gallery of Ireland)

earlier subscribers in order to meet the demand of later visitors to his studio. Consequently, to evade further investigation, Wheatley was reported to have fled back to England. He seems to have taken the painting with him, and eventually it found its way to Lotherton House, a stately home in Yorkshire in the custody of the city of Leeds, where it can be seen today. A detailed examination of the painting reveals some empty seats in the chamber, presumably where Wheatley had not had the time to add his next customer.

The women in the gallery had, therefore, paid for the privilege of being included in the painting. Caution is consequently called for in assuming that the painting reflected the reality of the occasion during the debate. There may well be some artistic (as well as commercial) licence involved. Nevertheless, we can confirm from other documentary sources that women's attendance in the Irish parliamentary gallery was a fairly commonplace event, particularly during important debates like that of 1780. During the debate on the constitutional legislation of 1782 Jonah Barrington estimated that there were over 400 women in the gallery. Contemporary accounts indicate that the front row of the gallery was usually reserved for 'ladies of the highest distinction'. Wheatley also, accurately, placed most of the women in his picture in the front section of the gallery.

The story of women's presence at Commons debates begins with the opening of the new parliamentary building in College Green in 1731. The new building was constructed to reflect the status and importance of the Irish parliament in the eighteenth century. It was also designed as a very public building in the centre of the most fashionable part of Dublin. Its layout and location indicated

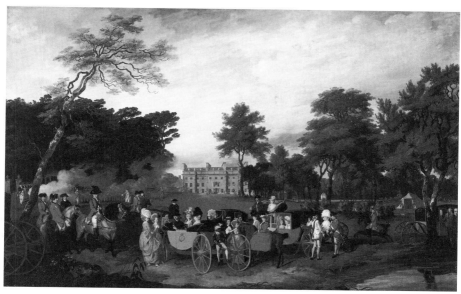

In this Wheatley painting of the Stafford family at Belan House, the dowager Lady Adleborough (mounted, in red) is dressed in a colonel's uniform. (Waddesdon, Rothschild Collection)

that it was intended to provide easy access for a select public. The main entrance off College Green, through a wide, columned open space, led into a public hall or foyer where people congregated during parliamentary sessions, often to submit petitions to be presented by sympathetic MPs to the Commons. The chamber of the House of Commons was, as Wheatley's painting indicates, surrounded by a wide public gallery, five feet wide, which could accommodate, according to one estimate, up to 700 people, with the seated front row reserved, as we have seen, for female visitors.

From its official opening in 1731 the parliament building was quickly integrated into the social scene of Dublin's Protestant élite. When the writer Mary Delany visited the city later in the same year, she spent the best part of a day in the building. She described how she and her party arrived at 11am and heard a dispute in the Commons' chamber concerning the outcome of an election. About 3pm they were brought chickens, ham and tongue, which they ate in the gallery, and, as she put it herself: At 4 o'clock the speaker adjourned the House 'till five. We then were conveyed, by some gentleman of our acquaintance, into the Usher of the Black Rod's room, where he had a good fire, and meat, tea, and bread and butter . . . When the House was assembled, we re-assumed our seats and staid till 8; loth was I to go away then'.

While Delany and her friends in the Protestant establishment no doubt viewed the proceedings in parliament as an interesting spectator sport, it is also important to consider the involvement of aristocratic women from landed families in Irish political life in the eighteenth century. It is a commonplace to assert that landownership and political power were closely linked in eighteenth-century Ireland, but the gender implications of this need also to be considered. Membership of a Protestant landed family automatically bestowed political influence, regardless of gender. Women as well as men canvassed for their families' parliamentary candidates and registered and lobbied voters on the family estate. Elizabeth Hastings, countess of Moira, and her daughter, Selina Rawdon, Lady Granard, for example, were both engaged in canvassing in the constituency of Granard in County Longford in the 1780s. One potential voter described how Lady Selina visited him and noted down in a pocketbook his request for a favour in return for securing his vote. This and other similar demands were usually related to securing appointments in the public service, and potential voters clearly believed that Lady Granard had access to political influence and could secure them a position.

The fact that membership of the Irish parliament was confined to Protestant candidates meant that parliamentary politics was dominated by a small community or group of families. And the smallness of the Irish political world also facilitated women's access to political influence. Throughout the century the House of Commons was a fairly incestuous institution, with many of the MPs being related to one another in complex family networks that often formed the basis for political alliances. In this inward-looking society, élite Protestant women had a politically influential role as marriage partners and intermediaries between the different factions.

It is likely, therefore, that when women attended the debates in the House of Commons they were doing so not just as passive supporters but often as people with considerable influence over the MPs in the chamber. And, of course, attendance in the gallery meant that they could keep an eye on their candidate's voting pattern. Jonah Barrington vividly described the impact that the women in the gallery had on the men in the chamber during the debate on the Act of Union:

> The gratification of the anti-unionists was unbounded: and as they walked deliberately in, one by one, to be counted, the eager spectators, ladies as well as gentlemen, leaning over the galleries, ignorant of the result, were panting with expectation. Lady Castlereagh, then one of the finest women of the court, appeared in the serjeant's box, palpitating for her husband's fate. The desponding appearance and fallen crests of the ministerial benches, and the exulting air of the opposition members as they entered were intelligible . . . A due sense of respect and decorum restrained the galleries within proper bounds; but a low cry of satisfaction from the female audience could not be prevented.

But it was not just as members of politically influential families that women gained access to the public world of politics. The prevailing ideology of colonial Ireland also encouraged the participation of women in political life. The emergence of patriot politics in eighteenth-century Ireland has been analysed by historians in detail, but the extent to which patriot politics facilitated women's involvement in the political process has not been appreciated. One of the most valuable contributions on the history of Irish patriotism in eighteenth-century Ireland has been made by Joep Leersen. He pointed out that until the 1770s Irish patriotism was primarily concerned with improving the economic conditions and trade of Ireland. The main way in which people could demonstrate their sense of patriotism was through contributing to the economic and social improvement of Ireland. So until the 1770s Irish patriotism was more about demonstrating a sense of civic awareness than railing against the evils of English colonial government. Patriotic writers and politicians promoted numerous projects to improve the trade and commerce of Ireland and to alleviate Irish poverty. A common theme in many proposals was the advancement of Irish-manufactured goods and produce. Patriotic Irish citizens could publicly demonstrate their patriotism through the purchase of Irish goods.

The importance of women in this patriotic endeavour was recognised by the pamphleteers. Many condemned the extravagance of wealthy women who imported the latest French and English fashions rather than support local Irish manufacturers. In 1722 Jonathan Swift specifically targeted such women in his pamphlet *A proposal that all the ladies and women of Ireland should appear constantly in Irish manufactures*. Swift's publication was followed by others encouraging women to buy Irish cloth and fashions. Successive wives of lord lieutenants attempted to set a good example by making the wearing of Irish cloth fashionable and issuing invitations to social events in Dublin Castle with instructions that only Irish-manufactured cloth was to be worn. Although such campaigns made little impact on the Irish textile industry, they did transform the wearing of Irish cloth into a symbol of virtuous patriotism. By the middle decades of the eighteenth century, élite women viewed the occasional purchase of Irish-produced textiles as an appropriate form of public charity. Patriotism thus gradually evolved into both a fashionable and a gender-inclusive sentiment.

The 'wear Irish' campaign was, however, more than simply a fashionable game for bored society women. It brought women into the public discourse, placed a value on their consumer power and therefore expanded their engagement with the public sphere. The patriotic Irish woman demonstrated her patriotism and her concern for the poor through the clothes that she wore.

By the 1770s Irish patriotism became more overtly political as the Volunteer campaign got under way and demanded greater political and economic freedom from Britain. The Volunteer demand for 'free trade' received widespread support in the late 1770s. The politicisation of the Volunteer movement coincided with a downturn in the Irish economy, which led to more calls on women to buy Irish-manufactured goods. By spring 1779 the demand for women to buy Irish cloth as an act of charity was transformed into a more overtly political gesture.

In North America, women had taken part in a boycott of British goods to demonstrate the colony's unhappiness with British control of its trade. The American boycott had been very effective, and the Irish Volunteers imitated the tactic by setting up a similar boycott movement in Ireland. Irish women were encouraged to follow the example of women in America. Newspaper editorials in 1779 were specifically addressed to women, encouraging them to become involved. For example, the *Freeman's Journal* in September 1779 addressed its editorial to the 'female patriots of Ireland' and encouraged Irish women to demonstrate their sense of patriotism in the same way as the women in America. And other editorials in the same and other newspapers carried similar addresses to women to become actively involved and to manifest their patriotism publicly. By the autumn of 1779, therefore, women who had initially supported the 'buy Irish' campaigns for charitable reasons found themselves at the centre of a more political and anti-English campaign. Women responded to these calls individually and collectively. In Dublin a group of women formed a non-importation association following a public meeting in April 1779, and later in the year a 'ladies' agreement' was left in a Dublin shop to be signed by women—according to the *Freeman's Journal*, it was signed by 'a great number of respectable names'.

In addition to their public support for the free trade campaign, women also attended Volunteer reviews in large numbers. It was common practice, for example, for officers' wives to appear on the reviewing stand, some dressed in the uniform of the regiment. The woman in the Volunteer uniform in Wheatley's painting of the House of Commons was undoubtedly the wife of an officer, possibly the man standing next to her. Women were also among the crowds who cheered and waved ribbons and handkerchiefs at the Volunteers when they marched through the streets of Dublin, and they appear to have also been admitted to the convention debates organised by the Volunteers in the Rotunda in 1783.

Francis Wheatley arrived in Dublin at the zenith of the popularity of the Volunteers and quickly assumed the role of unofficial artist of the movement. His paintings document the engagement of women with the Volunteers. Apart from his House of Commons painting, Wheatley's 'Volunteer review' also includes women in the windows overlooking College Green, wearing Volunteer colours, and one woman can just be distinguished dressed in a Volunteer uniform.

In another Wheatley painting, that of the Stafford family at Belan House in the midlands, the dowager Lady Adleborough is dressed in a colonel's uniform, while her daughter-in-law wears the uniform of her husband's regiment.

The Volunteers thus provided women with new ways of expressing their sense of patriotism in public, both at the level of the officers' wives and at the lower social level of women who participated in street protest. The Volunteer movement gave women a more visible political role than they had had before.

The new public role for women was, however, of short duration. By 1782 the Volunteers had been granted 'free trade' and some control over parliamentary legislation through the Declaration of 1782. In the 1780s the public debate moved on to the issue of parliamentary reform and the extension of the franchise. There was disagreement as to how many and which men should be enfranchised, but none of the contributors advocated granting women any formal role in the parliamentary process. The shift of focus to parliamentary reform reduced the political usefulness of women in political campaigns. By late 1783 the involvement of women in the Volunteer movement sparked a reaction against women's participation in public affairs, and the women who attended Volunteer reviews and the convention debates began to be mocked and scorned in Volunteer literature.

The United Irish movement that followed the Volunteers did not allot women a public role. Women were useful in the background, providing safe houses and backup support for men, but none of the United Irishmen advocated giving women a vote or more political responsibility. Some of the United Irishmen who visited France when they were negotiating for military aid wrote of their dislike of the women who participated in politics in Paris. While the Volunteer movement promoted the notion of the 'patriot woman', the United Irishmen did not promote the idea of the 'republican woman'. This was to come much later in the nineteenth century.

Finally, it is worth comparing women's engagement in politics in eighteenth-century Ireland with that of other countries. The access that élite women had to the Irish House of Commons was quite unusual, by the standards of the eighteenth century. In England in 1778, almost two years before Wheatley began his painting, the House of Commons banned women from the gallery. And in republican America after 1776 women neither voted for nor attended the debates in the inter-colonial assemblies. In France, women participated in the Revolution in 1789, particularly in the street protests in Paris. They were also initially admitted into the gallery of the National Assembly debates. But this eventually proved to be one step too far, as far as the revolutionary leaders were concerned. In 1794 women were formally prohibited from attending public debates in France. Meanwhile, back in Ireland, women continued to sit in the gallery of the Irish House of Commons—until its demise in 1801.

So, in terms of being involved in the politics of the parliament, it could be argued that women in Ireland had a more visible profile than women in other countries. The evolution of patriot politics in the 1770s also expanded the opportunities for Irish women to become involved in the public sphere. Linda Colley has suggested that it was not until the wars of the 1790s that it became socially acceptable for women in England to demonstrate their sense of patriotism in a public fashion. It could be argued, therefore, that the colonial circumstances in Ireland and the smallness of its political community facilitated a stronger political role for élite women in Ireland than in England. A more favourable comparison can be made between women in Ireland and in the other British colony, in North America. Historians have long recognised the role that women played in the American Revolution through the boycott of British goods. Women in Ireland, particularly in Dublin, were, arguably, as actively involved in the Volunteer campaign as women in North America were in the boycott campaign of the Revolution. Historians have just not recognised it.

Chapter Five

'Better without the ladies': The Royal Irish Academy and the admission of women members

Clare O'Halloran

This topic suggested itself while I was studying Irish antiquarianism during the Enlightenment. I was investigating the Royal Irish Academy (RIA) and the scholarly and political élite who were central to its establishment in 1785 as the national body for the promotion of 'science, polite literature and antiquities'. I was looking at the scholarly activities of the only woman active in antiquarian research at the time of the Academy's foundation: the well-connected but impecunious Charlotte Brooke (daughter of the playwright Henry Brooke), who produced the first major collection of translations of Gaelic poetry into English, *Reliques of Irish poetry* (1789). While in particular financial difficulty in 1787, she petitioned the council of the newly formed academy to be appointed housekeeper for their recently acquired premises. (There was, of course, no question of a woman becoming a member, but in any case, her desire was not for recognition but rather for basic shelter.) A year later, the council made a decision to appoint its official clerk and mace-bearer (who happened to be a brother of the poet Oliver Goldsmith) to the post of housekeeper with 'an allowance of £40 per annum and coals'. Like the premier British scientific institution, the Royal Society of London, the Irish academicians preferred to keep theirs a male-only space, even in terms of employees. As for Charlotte Brooke, she had to shift for herself and died in poverty in 1791.

On the other hand, offering honorary membership to internationally renowned women scholars could be used to signal the status of the RIA as a fully participating institute in international scientific culture. Thus, the academy made the acclaimed English mathematician and science writer Mary Somerville an honorary member in 1834, one year in advance of the Royal Astronomical Society. In 1838 the astronomer Caroline Herschel (who had been honoured at the same time as Mary Somerville by the Royal Astronomical Society) was offered honorary membership by the RIA. Part of the attraction of honouring Somerville and Herschel may well have been that they were foreign female luminaries, and thus there was no danger that they could lay claim to occupy the space or privileges of full academicians. Like the Royal Society installing a bust of Mary Somerville in the Great Hall while not allowing her to set foot there, the Irish academicians could recognise international female achievement in their own way without threatening the male-only boundaries of their space.

In 1842 the academy elected the first of its two Irish female honorary members. This was Maria Edgeworth, the best-known (male or female) Irish novelist of the day, whose father, Richard Lovell Edgeworth, had been a founder member of the academy and one of the famous Lunar Society of Birmingham members before he moved to Ireland. The minutes of the Academy record that she was elected 'by acclamation', but it could be said that they had waited until almost the last minute to honour her—given that she was 74 in 1842, and with her creative years behind her.

We do not know how Edgeworth viewed her belated recognition by the premier institution in Ireland charged with promoting 'polite literature'. We have, however, some insight into her views on such male-only bodies from her writings. In her *Letters for literary ladies*, an early work of 1795 which advocated the proper education of women for, amongst other reasons, the improvement of family life, she argued that if men 'meet with conversation suited to their taste at home, they will not be driven to clubs . . . from which ladies are to be excluded'.

Some 40 years later, and four years before being made an honorary academician, her friend the mathematician William Rowan Hamilton, as newly elected president of the RIA, consulted her as to how best the Academy could advance 'the interests of polite literature' in Ireland. She used the opportunity to suggest opening the Academy to women, albeit in a limited way:

> [Y]our admitting ladies to your evening parties would be advantageous—I think provided you do commence those parties for the ladies late enough for their fashion and so give your gentlemen time enough to themselves after dinner for conversation and discussions which might be uninteresting to the fair visitors or in which they might possibly be *de trop*.

As Edgeworth explained in a later letter, what she had in mind here was for the academy to create in Dublin a version of the celebrated informal *conversaziones* or *soirées* held regularly in London by the science writer Jane Marcet (a close friend of Edgeworth's), where, as she told Hamilton, she 'had the pleasure and advantage of meeting all [Marcet's] scientific and literary friends who used to give her half an hour [on] their way to or from the meetings of the Royal Society', and she assured him that such events were 'very agreeable to men of both science and literature'. Here Edgeworth was anticipating, by a decade or two, the establishment by most learned bodies of at least annual *conversaziones*, through which the middle-class appetite for science and the arts was catered for by evenings of public lectures, music and exhibitions in the premises of the societies.

Hamilton, however, politely but firmly rejected Edgeworth's suggestion, arguing first that it was 'physically impossible to give accomodation [*sic*] to ladies', owing to the small size of the academy's meeting room, and secondly, that their regular meetings involved the discussion of 'questions of legislation and finance' and that while it was 'comparatively easy to desire male visitors to withdraw . . . it would be hard to ask ladies to do so'. His solution was to maintain the men-only format, with the hope that their meetings would afterwards generate discussion 'in the more graceful circle of the drawing-room, and with the advantage of that animation and polish which belongs to good female society'. Edgeworth's response to this patronising rebuff was wonderfully ironic in its apparent feminine meekness:

> I am rather sorry that you wasted a page upon a suggestion of mine which you have completely convinced me could not be carried into effect, and which . . . at the moment I put it on paper . . . seemed to me to be too lady-like a scheme—to smell too much of the drawing room if not of the shop—you are certainly as you have proved to me physically and morally, and intellectually better without the ladies—without turning your academical questions and business into *conversazione* babble.

Almost twenty years later, the academy held an elaborate *conversazione* during the 1857 meeting of the British Association for the Advancement of Science (BAAS) in Dublin, taking over the neighbouring public rooms and gardens of the lord mayor's residence for the purpose. Clearly the problem of space could be overcome for the BAAS, if not for the 'ladies' of Dublin.

When the campaign for university education for women was finally successful (from the early 1880s the Queen's Colleges began to admit women students, with Trinity College Dublin bringing up the rear in 1904), it was inevitable that a woman would be nominated for full membership of the RIA. The admission of women was on the agendas of many learned societies at around this time. In 1903 the Linnaean Society in London resolved the issue in favour of admitting women by obtaining a supplementary charter which inserted the words 'without distinction of sex' into the clauses relating to the election of fellows. But in 1902, when the Royal Society was forced to consider the nomination of the first woman fellow, the legal advice was that their charter definitely precluded married women joining and very probably single women also.

Since the RIA had always modeled itself closely on the Royal Society, it was perhaps inevitable that when, in 1910, it was faced with the first nomination of a woman member (referred to only as 'a [widow] lady') this negative decision would be influential. At a council meeting in February 1910 there seems to have been some support for the nomination and the principle it would have established, as a motion was introduced to accept the nomination under the usual procedures and to put it to a ballot of members. An amendment to this was passed, however, to defer the issue until legal advice was obtained. Writing the following September, the Academy's solicitor relied heavily in his opinion on that supplied to the Royal Society in 1902 and advised that under the current charter women could not lawfully be admitted to membership.

There the matter rested until 1919, when Westminster passed the Sex Disqualification (Removal) Act, article 1 of which stated, among other things, that a 'person shall not be disqualified by sex or marriage from . . . admission to any incorporated society (whether incorporated by royal charter or otherwise)'. A number of learned societies in the two islands were slow to react to this unambiguously enabling act, but the Irish academies had, perhaps, the excuse that the act came at a time of political and military upheaval in the country, just as the War of Independence got under way. The new Irish Free State that came into existence in 1922 gave a clear (but, as it turned out, misleading) signal of progressive tendencies in terms of women's rights by granting the vote to all citizens 'without distinction of sex' at the age of 21 (30 remained the qualifying age for British women until 1928). British statute and common law up to 1920 continued to have force in Ireland, unless or until amended or repealed by the Irish government, so that the 1919 Sex Disqualification (Removal) Act remained valid.

In 1927, however, as part of a backlash against women's rights, the Irish Free State government amended the 1919 Sex Disqualification (Removal) Act to abolish women's duty to undertake jury service, requiring them to opt in should they wish to serve. Given the government's determination to reassert legally the traditional place of women in the home rather than in public life, the status of the 1919 act was felt to be in doubt throughout the 1920s, and this provides one possible explanation for the reluctance of the RIA to accept the legal position and open its membership to women. When, in 1930, the council finally sought legal opinion on the question in the light of the 1919 act, their solicitor advised that 'the charter of the academy must now be read as applying to women as well as men' but that this legislation did not provide for the appointment of women as officers of the Academy.

So in 1931 the RIA, like the other reluctant learned societies of the two islands, had to bow to the inevitable: the president, according to the council minutes, 'made a statement informing the council that legal opinion had been taken on the question of the eligibility of women for membership of the Academy. The opinion given was that in the existing state of the law women are eligible.' As with the Royal Society (and many other national academies of science), however, the first female members were not elected until after World War II. In 1949 four women were admitted, two scientists and two in the humanities: Sheila Power (later Tinney), lecturer and later Associate Professor of Mathematical Physics (Quantum Theory), UCD; Phyllis Clinch, lecturer and later holder of the chair in Botany, UCD; archaeologist and art historian Françoise Henry, UCD; and Eleanor Knott, Professor of Celtic Languages, TCD.

Between 1950 and 1957 seven more women were elected (one per year), three in science and four in the humanities, making a total of eleven women members. Thirty years later, in 1987, the figure still stood at eleven, out of a total membership of 250 (or just over 5%). (It was at this time that I witnessed the members' procession containing one solitary female.) Since then there has been a concerted effort to elect more women, bringing the total, as of 2011, to 56 female members. The overall membership has increased to 455, however, so the proportion of women has only increased to 12.3%. Most are in the humanities (45 in total), reflecting, in part, the global scarcity of women in the sciences. Indeed, the gender balance is likely to continue this glacial progress towards equality as a result of a decision to concentrate recruitment in the information technology and engineering fields, which could be seen in the 2010 and 2011 intakes, in which just nine out of 48 new members were female.

Yet when one turns one's attention to the sizeable administrative staff who run the extensive research and publishing programmes now under the academy's remit, the gender balance is reversed: it is overwhelmingly female (although with disproportionately more men in senior positions). Thus, more than 200 years after her fruitless petition, Charlotte Brooke might now readily find space in that part of the Royal Irish Academy, but this hardly seems like sufficient progress after two centuries.

Chapter Six

'Women of the pave': Prostitution in Ireland

Maria Luddy

Thousands of women working as prostitutes roamed the streets of the towns and cities of Ireland in the nineteenth and early twentieth centuries. While there was a common belief that prostitution was an inevitable feature of life, especially where military garrisons existed, as long as prostitutes remained out of the public eye they were tolerated. It was most often their visibility that caused anxiety in the wider public. Prostitutes were believed to be the main source of venereal disease infection, and prostitution itself was believed to be contagious. In 1809 the women prisoners confined for debt in the Four Courts Marshalsea in Dublin, fearing moral and physical contagion, complained about having to mix with 'women of the town (some from the very flags [streets])'.

There are few, if any, reliable statistics on the extent of prostitution. The two best sources are the police statistics for the Dublin Metropolitan District from 1838 to 1919, and the criminal and judicial statistics from 1863 (covering the entire country). The figures account for arrests and convictions of women accused of soliciting; they do not record the number of re-arrests. Since many women were arrested dozens of times within any one year, these figures do not tally with the numbers of women operating as prostitutes. They also fluctuate widely—giving the impression that prostitution is diminishing or increasing—but in a way not backed up by other evidence. On the other hand, it is unlikely that every prostitute was arrested. Sarah Wilson was imprisoned 40 times on various dates between 2 September 1875 and 2 August 1877. Committed by magistrates at Newbridge, the Curragh and Naas, her offences included trespass, being drunk and disorderly, and obstructing the footpath. Her sentences ranged from three days to three months. Similarly, a woman confined to Grangegorman prison for five years for larceny in 1885 was recorded in the register as a prostitute, and at the age of 44 had accumulated 93 previous convictions.

Such statistics give us a general idea of where and when the police were most vigilant in arresting prostitutes. The Dublin Metropolitan Police (DMP)

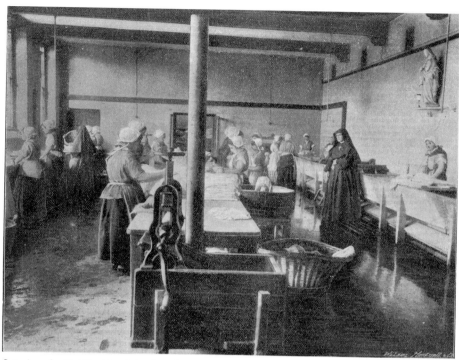

Interior of a Dublin Magdalen laundary in the 1890s. (British Library)

statistics show that 2,849 arrests were made in 1838, increasing yearly to a maximum of 4,784 in 1856 and decreasing to 1,672 in 1877, fluctuating around the 1,000 mark from then to the 1890s and reaching a low of 494 in 1899. In the twentieth century the highest number of arrests, consequent on the introduction of the Criminal Law Amendment Act, is in 1912, with 1,067 detentions, and then the arrest figures gradually decrease to a low of 198 by 1919. If we look at the figures for the entire country, we find that in 1863 (and these figures include Dublin) there were 3,318 arrests for prostitution. Leinster consistently had the highest number of arrests, and Connacht the least. Galway City rarely features, but prostitution certainly existed there. The 1851 census listed 27 prostitutes and brothel-keepers in County Galway (four in the city) that go unrecorded in the crime statistics. In 1881, when no arrests were returned for Galway City, a policeman stationed there described a brothel in Middle Street as 'the worst house in Ireland'.

The DMP suggested that there were 1,630 prostitutes in Dublin in 1838; by 1890 that figure had declined to 436. A number of women worked in brothels, though they did not necessarily live in these establishments. Brothels, recorded in police statistics as of either a 'superior' or 'inferior' type, were most common

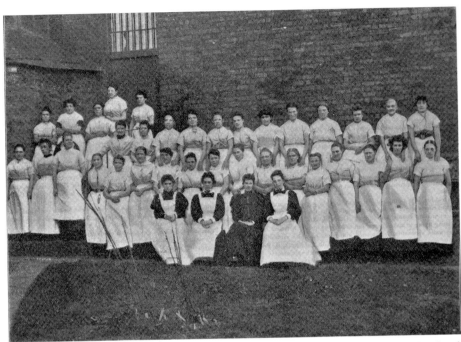

A group of inmates in the Dublin Female Penitentiary, Berkeley Place, North Circular Road, Dublin, 15 April 1897. (British Library)

in Dublin but also existed in other towns and cities. In 1842 there were 1,287 brothels in Dublin. During the Famine years the number of brothels in the city hovered between 330 and 419, with more than 1,300 women working from them. By 1894 there were 74 brothels operating openly in Dublin and an average of three women worked from each of them. The infamous Mrs Mack, who appears in the 'Nighttown' episode of *Ulysses*, kept a brothel at 85 Lower Tyrone Street in the heart of the red-light (Monto) district of Dublin. She was so well known that the area was often referred to as 'Macktown'. The 1901 census records that Mack had five 'lodgers', ranging in age from 21 to 27, listed as dressmaker, housekeeper, waitress, milliner and lace-maker. Also listed was a servant and a widow aged 32, who probably looked after the women. The 'lodgers' were all literate and unmarried; two were from England, while the rest came from outside Dublin. Eliza Mack herself was 50 at this time, a widow who had been born in Cork City. She was described by Oliver St John Gogarty as having 'a brick-red face, on which avarice was written like a hieroglyphic, and a laugh like a guffaw in hell'.

The police were slow to close brothels, believing that this spread the problem into new areas by dispersing the women. Prostitution was often the resort of

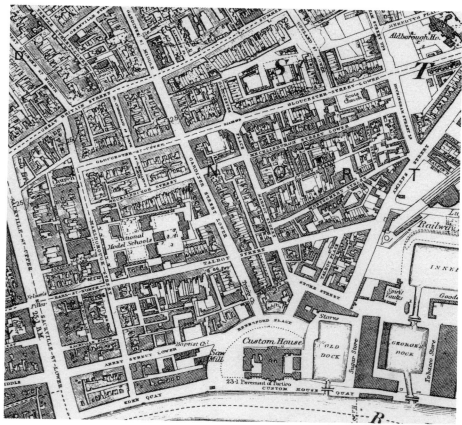

The 'Monto' in 1876. (Ordnance Survey of Ireland)

the desperate in a country that offered limited opportunities to women and where a change in economic circumstances, such as the loss of employment or desertion by a spouse or breadwinner, plunged many women into economic crisis. Evidence from the Poor Inquiry of 1836 suggests that unmarried mothers who could not get the putative fathers to support them and the children were 'in some instances driven . . . to prostitution as a mode of support'. Susanna Price took to prostitution and crime to support herself when her soldier husband was overseas. In 1840 she was sentenced to seven years' transportation for larceny. Catherine Grady, 'a notoriously improper character and public nuisance', pleaded guilty to theft in Kilkenny in 1846 and was transported for seven years. The reporter commented that it was a 'happy riddance for the city'. Bridget Hayes, who was transported for larceny in 1848, pleaded that she had been seduced by a young man who cast her off and that she 'had to pursue a wicked life to keep herself from starvation'.

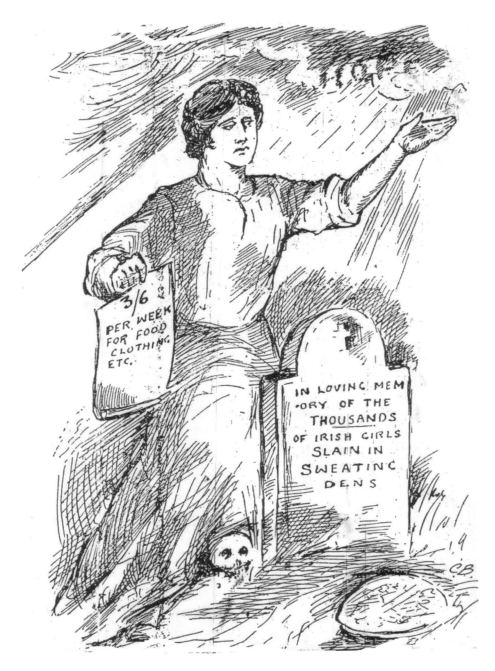

White Slavery in Dublin !

'White Slavery in Dublin' *(The Irish Worker, 25 May 1912).*

Prostitutes were most often charged with theft, being drunk and disorderly, vagrancy and sometimes murder. When convicted of soliciting the general sentence was a fine or, in default of payment, two weeks or longer in prison. In Kilkenny a prostitute who stole £200 from a farmer got six months with hard labour in 1871. The judge had little sympathy for the victim, observing that married men should not be 'going about drinking with abandoned females'. It is also evident that many newspaper reporters used some of these court cases as a way to amuse their readers. For instance, two women who lived in a hovel in Ennis were charged with not paying their landlord rent. In evidence it emerged that both women, Fanny Crowe and Bridget Hogan, were 'prostitutes of the most infamous character' and considered a nuisance to the entire neighbourhood. Fanny Crowe was described as 'a masculine looking woman with a Connacht accent'. Crowe, when asked by a solicitor if she was not a 'quiet, mild and respectable woman', answered, to the delight of the court, 'I think it would be very hard for you to find a woman that you'd get the three in'.

In the cities, renaming streets associated with prostitution was relatively common. Anderson's Row in Belfast, noted as an area of immorality, became Millfield Place in December 1860, though this did not improve its reputation. In 1885 Lower Temple Street, Dublin, became Hill Street in consequence of a memorial to the Corporation from a number of inhabitants who 'had suffered serious deterioration in the value of [their] property' as certain houses in the lower end of the street were occupied by 'immoral characters'. In 1888 Dublin Corporation renamed Mecklenburgh Street Tyrone Street to please the respectable working-class residents of the area.

As the nineteenth century progressed, prostitution in Dublin had become more geographically confined. After the 1870s women began to move into cheaper accommodations available in the Lower Mecklenburgh Street area. The evidence of the Revd Robert Conlan to a commission on housing in 1885 revealed that brothels were extending into the district. He observed that some of the houses were regular bad houses, but that in the case of tenement houses 'bad people who would carry on the same trade would take a flat', so that brothels in this area were now to be found in tenement houses that also contained respectable families.

As early as 1837 this area was noted for its 'great number of destitute poor, [and] dissolute and depraved characters' of both sexes. The Mecklenburgh/ Montgomery district of the city, north-east of the Custom House, marked the infamous 'Monto' district. By 1911 the renaming of streets in this area saw Waterford Street and Railway Street remaining notorious. While Tyrone Street was the most infamous street in the area, with a considerable number of brothels, the adjoining streets, Foley Street, Montgomery Street, Mabbot

Street, Beaver Street, Purdon Street, Elliott Place, Faithful Place, Uxbridge and Nickleby, were almost as disreputable. In this area was located the famous 'Becky Cooper's' (immortalised as Bella Cohen's in the 'Circe' episode of Joyce's *Ulysses*) and Mrs Mack's, located at 85 Tyrone Street. Halliday Sutherland recalled that in 1904, as a medical student in Dublin, he had walked one evening down Tyrone Street. He observed that 'in no other capital of Europe have I seen its equal. It was a street of Georgian houses and each one was a brothel. On the steps of every house women and girls dressed in everything from evening dress to a nightdress stood or sat.'

While it was to the 'Monto' area that prostitutes in Dublin had been gradually confined from the 1880s, this did not mean that prostitution did not exist or was less obvious in other parts of the city. Sackville Street (now O'Connell Street) was a principal promenading ground for prostitutes, and many were also to be found in the Phoenix Park, St Stephen's Green and around the dock area. A police commissioner reported that prior to 1922 prostitution was mainly confined to a particular area stretching from Summerhill to Talbot Street and from Marlborough Street to the Five Lamps at the junction of Amiens Street and Portland Row.

Women who worked as prostitutes left themselves open to violence and abuse. Mary Flanagan, for instance, an 'exceedingly juvenile cyprian', appeared before the court in Ennis in October 1845. She alleged that a client, Francis Kelly, had enticed her into a field and raped her at knifepoint over a period of three hours. Kelly was later acquitted when Flanagan refused to identify him. In Limerick, Mary Carmody, who admitted she had been a prostitute for four years, accused a young man of raping her. Her assailant, who said she was 'a prostitute and she was bound to go with him', told police she had taken a shilling and then told him to go to hell. Despite his claim he was convicted, as was a soldier whose excuse for raping a prostitute was that he had no money. Three men had attempted to drown a prostitute by throwing her off Pope's Quay in Cork in 1839. A number of these women attempted suicide. Kathleen Dolan did so by jumping into the river in Galway, stating that she 'would not put up with all the warrants and imprisonments'. A small number appear to have been committed to lunatic asylums. 'K.D.' was confined to Ballinasloe Asylum with 'dementia', having been imprisoned for attempting suicide. Ellen Byrne, a 26-year-old prostitute from Dublin, committed infanticide after being refused entry to the workhouse. Found guilty but insane, she was sent in 1893 to Dundrum Mental Hospital, where she died within the year.

Whatever their treatment by the courts or the public, prostitutes were not without some forms of resistance. It was a common practice for women to change their names to confuse the authorities. They formed a generally mobile population, migrating to towns and cities. With some groups of prostitutes there was also solidarity, seen particularly in the case of the 'Wrens' of the Curragh. It was noted by a number of magistrates that when arrested the women were often 'very violent, and threw themselves down and refuse to walk'. Sometimes the women committed crimes to go to jail and receive medical attention or a respite from their harsh life. For instance, in 1846 Mary Murphy pleaded guilty to breaking the windows of the mayor's office in Kilkenny in order to be imprisoned.

By the end of the nineteenth century geographical limits were placed on where brothels and prostitutes might operate unhindered. Prostitutes, however, still roamed much more freely than the public or authorities wished. By the early twentieth century Irish nationalists argued that prostitution and venereal disease were symptoms of the British presence in Ireland and that it was only with Irish independence that they would disappear. Apparent rises in the rates of illegitimacy, venereal diseases and sexual crime in the 1920s suggest the simple-mindedness of that view.

Chapter Seven

A sexual revolution in the west of Ireland? Workhouses and illegitimacy in post-Famine Ireland

Paul Gray and Liam Kennedy

ew places suffered more severely from a combination of eviction and famine than Kilrush in County Clare and its surrounding districts in the mid-nineteenth century. Only Skibbereen in south-west Cork and a few other parishes in the west of Ireland are likely to have experienced a comparable degree of human misery.

But Kilrush has a further claim on our attention, and that is the apparent surge in illegitimate births in the two decades after the Great Famine. By 1864 these accounted for one in ten of all births recorded in the baptism register of the Catholic parish of Kilrush, a remarkably high proportion for mid-Victorian Ireland. Before the Famine the ratio was barely one in a hundred in most years. The spectacular and sustained rise in recorded illegitimate births might suggest a revolution in sexual mores in this remote town and its hinterland. This is all the more surprising in that the west of Ireland is generally considered to have had a low incidence of bastardy, to use the quaint demographer's term.

So, what was going on? One possibility is that the Famine itself and the associated evictions may have served to push up illegitimacy. The argument might run as follows. In the cauldron of suffering that was Kilrush at the end of the 1840s, it hardly seems far-fetched to imagine that some poor women bartered sex for immediate comfort, either in the form of food or simply companionship and evanescent pleasure. Food shortage also opened up possibilities for the sexual exploitation of women. More typically, perhaps, those who found themselves with child might conform to the demographer's notion of 'illegitimacy as marriage frustrated'. In better times, the putative father might have been obliged to honour his responsibilities.

But these were not normal times. The collapse of the economy of the potato-eaters, the decimation of family and kinfolk, and the advent of mass emigration meant that abandonment was a strategic alternative for the restless and

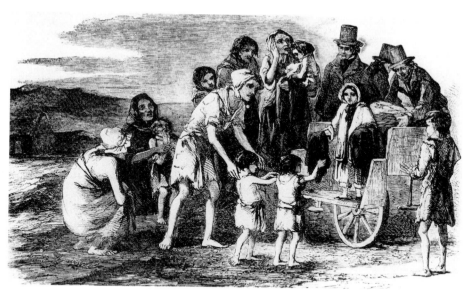

Miss Kennedy, seven-year-old daughter of Capt. Kennedy, Poor Law inspector of the Kilrush Union, distributing clothing to the destitute of the area. (Illustrated London News).

irresponsible male. So, in desperate times, the orchestration of social pressures was less easily accomplished, and the vulnerable and the trusting—particularly if they had suffered the loss through death or migration of supportive family or kinfolk—were more likely to end up carrying the baby alone.

It is the case that illegitimacy in Kilrush rose during the Famine and in its immediate aftermath, but the Famine effect is likely to have been short-term rather than long-term in nature. Another possibility hinges on the status of Kilrush as a port town—sometimes associated with prostitution and illegitimacy—and as the gateway to the growing holiday resorts of west Clare, in particular Kilkee on the Atlantic coastline.

Indeed, a visitor to Kilkee in 1855 complained that this tourist resort was 'infested by a number of unfortunate women, who disturb the inhabitants and visitors at night'. Some must have enjoyed having their nights disturbed because, despite a public condemnation from the pulpit of the Catholic Church, the problem persisted. Two of these roving women, described as 'young ladies from Kilrush', were assaulted by the local priest, Fr McMahon, who was subsequently fined one shilling and costs for his pains. The Clare historian Ciaran Ó Murchadha (in a private communication), informed us of the sex trade being supplemented seasonally, to coincide with the tourist trade, by prostitutes from Limerick city. Thus, it seems, not only tourists but also prostitutes circulated along a Limerick–Kilrush/Kilkee axis.

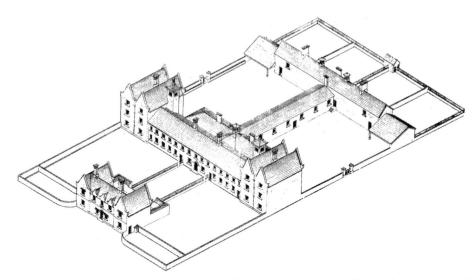

Plan of a workhouse, 1839 – while unmarried and pregnant women suffered stigmatisation and degradation under the workhouse system, men appear to have largely escaped notice or sanction. (House of Commons Parliamentary Papers)

Still, this can only be a small part of the story, not least in view of the seasonal and migratory nature of the trade. Another speculative possibility is that Kilrush was somehow nurturing, to use Peter Lalett's words, a bastardy-prone sub-society. But of the 211 mothers recorded as giving birth to children outside wedlock in the quarter-century after the Famine, only eighteen per cent were 'repeaters' (bearers of more than one illegitimate offspring).

To take an example or two, Mary Giffin had illegitimate children baptised in August 1858, August 1861, September 1863 and September 1868. Then there was Margaret Byrnes, whose illegitimate children were baptised in June 1859, March 1861, August 1863 and May 1865. But these were the exception. Most single mothers did not repeat the experience of bearing a child outside of marriage.

The real explanation turns out to be much simpler than any of the preceding lines of interpretation would suggest. A more detailed examination of the Catholic baptismal register for Kilrush reveals that almost two out of every three births for the period 1850–75 were to women from the workhouse. The Kilrush workhouse served the whole union, not just the parish of Kilrush. If these workhouse births (baptisms) are excluded, then the numbers attributable to Kilrush fall back towards the more conventional levels of a west of Ireland town.

Thus the apparently inflated levels of illicit sexuality in Kilrush after the Famine arise primarily from a quirk of registration rather than from a radical shift in sexual behaviour on the part of Clare men and Clare women. This in

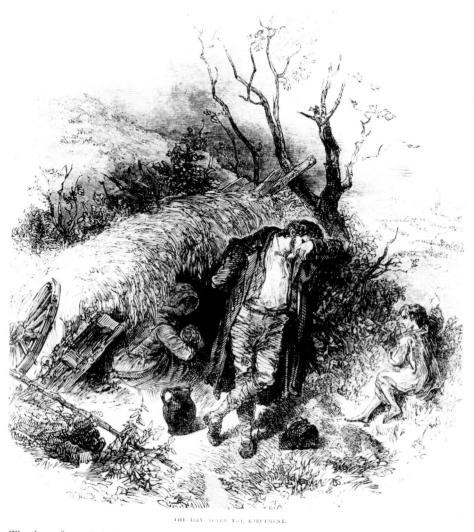

THE DAY AFTER THE EJECTMENT.

The day after eviction' – few places suffered more severely from a combination of eviction and famine than Kilrush. (Illustrated London News).

turn raises wider questions about the validity of parish register information on bastardy, not just for Ireland but for other societies where the institutionalised provision of welfare might affect the recording of illegitimate births.

What of the lives of these unmarried mothers, who increasingly used the workhouse as a lying-in hospital? Unfortunately, indoor relief registers for Kilrush, which would give some detail of the individual lives of unmarried mothers, have not survived. The indoor relief registers for the Rathdrum and

Shillelagh Poor Law unions (situated in the main in County Wicklow) have somehow survived, however, and provide poignant cameos of unmarried mothers and their children. Some of these individuals appear to have merited only a few lines. For instance, Mary Donnelly, a 22-year-old servant from Arklow, was admitted to Rathdrum workhouse on 16 August 1850. Heavily pregnant, she gave birth to Thomas on 6 September and left with him ten days later. She does not appear to have returned to the house. Ellen Power entered Rathdrum on 18 February 1851. She was a 24-year-old charwoman, described as from the 'union' and therefore most likely homeless. Her daughter was born on 27 March 1851 and conveyed from the workhouse on 8 August 1851, apparently without her mother, who left on the 14th of that month. Eliza Ashton, a 22-year-old servant, arrived in Rathdrum workhouse on 17 September 1850, leaving again a week later. She was described as from the 'union'. On 6 October she was admitted sick, and less than a week later Thomas was born. Both mother and child left on 26 October. She apparently did not return to the house again.

If some unmarried mothers left little trace in the workhouse record, others made many appearances. For example, Eliza Geoghan used the Rathdrum workhouse 23 times between 27 August 1850 and 2 June 1862. During that time her son John was born on 21 December 1850. Eliza was described as a 25-year-old garden worker. Mother and child left the house on 24 February 1851. Both entered the workhouse again, John being taken away on 24 June, a month before his mother left. Nothing more is known of John. Eliza, however, returned to the workhouse, pregnant, on 19 February 1854, and Dennis was born just over a week later. Both mother and child left on 23 June 1854. Eliza and Dennis entered the house three more times between June 1854 and April 1856. On their last visit on 23 September 1855, however, Dennis was to die, on 9 April 1856. Eliza left on 18 April. She gave birth to no more children in the workhouse but returned many times, spending the winters of 1856 and 1857 there. Over most of the twelve years she resided in the electoral division of Dunganstown East, changing her residence to another townland only twice. On her last two visits, however, she was described as from 'union Rathdrum', most likely signalling homelessness and increased destitution. She was mostly described as a 'servant', but also at times as a 'charwoman' and 'garden worker', and on the penultimate visit, of those surveyed, she was 'infirm' and apparently unemployed.

Another vignette is that of Jane Allen, who was to use Rathdrum workhouse on 34 occasions between 17 September 1850 and 13 March 1863. Jane Allen, aged 26, servant, arrived in Rathdrum workhouse on 17 September 1850 and gave birth to John on 19 October. John was taken away on 6 June 1851 and his mother left four days later. Nothing more is known of John. Jane was to have three more children: Eliza (30 July 1852), born in the house, Ellen (1856), born outside the house, and James (8 September 1861), born in the house. Jane stayed in Dunganstown South or Dunganstown West electoral divisions, occasionally changing townlands. Sometimes she and her children would stay for a number of months. On other occasions they stayed a matter of days. Although during her earlier stays in the workhouse she was referred to as a servant, for most of the times that she used the workhouse she was described as a charwoman. Perhaps more intriguingly, her marital status changed during the period. Although she was single for the period up to February 1861, she is described as 'married' during her stay in February/March 1861. On her next admittance, in August 1861, she is described as 'single'. In the meantime, her children were admitted as 'deserted' in March 1861, leaving in June 1861. The family was reunited in August 1861, and they entered the house five more times; on each occasion Jane is described as married, though one must wonder if she was not in fact a deserted wife, or perhaps intermittently so.

Such portraits help to bring out the perilous existence of the unmarried mother. Viewed from one angle, the workhouse could be seen as a resource, the use of which was one element in a larger strategy of survival on the part of the poor, including unmarried mothers. In this sense, we can speak of the unmarried mother possessing a degree of agency. But the balance in mid- and late Victorian Ireland would seem to lie in the opposite direction, that of desperation and choices of an extremely circumscribed kind. Over much of rural Ireland—the situation may have varied more within urban and industrialised Ulster—unmarried mothers faced religious, family and community hostility, and an unsympathetic, sometimes punitive system of welfare provision. Bastard-bearers were ground between the wheels of civil society and the state.

Little is known of the fate of illegitimate children. The register for Shillelagh affords the occasional glimpse. Eliza Pearson, aged four, was 'found at the door' of Shillelagh workhouse and was 'deserted by mother Anne'. She was taken into the workhouse on 19 June 1850 and left on 10 April 1856. Thomas Dwier, aged five, described as 'bastard', was admitted on 29 February 1852. His mother had been transported and he was 'destitute without food'. There is no record of his departure from the workhouse. Finally, Bridget Nugent was nine when she was 'deserted by father'. A 'deserted bastard', she had 'no friends nor residences' and was admitted on 10 January 1851, leaving on 28 July 1855. Here is one of the few instances where a male is mentioned in connection with an illegitimate child. While unmarried and pregnant women suffered stigmatisation and degradation under both the workhouse system and in the larger society, men appear to have largely escaped notice or sanction.

Thus Thurles union, in its reply to a Poor Law Commissioners' circular regarding moral classification, revealed the unfairness in gender terms of a system that singled out female morality in the workhouse, observing that 'no classification in this respect has been made at the male side'. If there are few clues as to the unmarried mothers in Kilrush who graced the parish records, albeit briefly, even less is known of those shadowy but potent figures of males who set women on a downward course to vilification, destitution and disgrace.

One of the ironies of the history of the Irish workhouse is that it could itself become a site for 'immoral behaviour', despite the rules and regimentation that governed these grim institutions. The minutes for the Kilrush union for 1853 reveal that the master and the matron of the workhouse had been accused of immorality. The accused were, however, later acquitted. According to the rules and regulations of the Poor Law system, women and men were to be strictly segregated within the penal institution of the workhouse. But in 1853 the master reported, no doubt with some trepidation:

> I beg to report to the board that Mr Nolan the resident apothecary informed me on Sunday last that a pauper woman named Kate Quinn who has been in this house for a long time was pregnant. On enquiry it would appear that a pauper man named John Griffin who is also in the house for a long period is the father. Kate Quinn left the workhouse on the 15th inst. Griffin also took his discharge on the 17th inst.

The Poor Law guardians were not amused: 'It is much to be regretted that such an evil should occur and the guardians conceive that there must be much neglect on the part of the officers in charge'.

The workhouse system was the subject of much contemporary and later criticism. It certainly bore down heavily on its inmates, both in terms of physical hardship and stigmatisation. But it needs to be recognised that it also furnished a safety net for the single mother in her battle for survival in the increasingly hostile moral climate of later Victorian Ireland and the 'Devotional Revolution'. The history of labour exploitation and repression, and sometimes outright cruelty, associated with the later Magdalene asylums, run by Irish Catholic nuns, suggests that there was no easy way out of the trap of unmarried motherhood, either in pre-independence or post-independence Ireland.

Chapter Eight

'Most vicious and refractory girls': The reformatories at Ballinasloe and Monaghan

Geraldine Curtin

On 2 July 1883, fifteen-year-old Bridget Carroll arrived at the Sparka's Lake reformatory in County Monaghan to serve the remainder of a sentence that had been imposed on her four years earlier. She had been tried at Loughrea petty sessions in September 1879 on a charge that she 'did threaten to stab Anne Flynn'. She was found guilty and sentenced to a short term of imprisonment, followed by five years in a reformatory in Ballinasloe, County Galway. This reformatory, which had been her home for nearly four years, was now closing, and she had made the long journey to Monaghan to serve out her sentence under the supervision of the St Louis sisters.

The foundress of the Monaghan school was Genevieve Beale, a Catholic convert. She had been born Priscilla Beale to Protestant, possibly Quaker, parents in London in 1822. Her father was a property developer and speculator and it was the failure of his business that led Priscilla to take up a position with a family in Cork. While there, she became acquainted with Fr Mathew, the 'apostle of temperance', and Ellen Woodlock, who, though a Cork native, had been living at Juilly in France. When Priscilla converted, Mrs Woodlock encouraged her to enter the convent founded by the Abbé Bautain at Juilly. She was professed there in October 1848 and became Sr Genevieve. She trained as a teacher and became superior of the newly established St Louis convent in Paris. Priscilla Beale was not the only young woman to make the journey from Ireland to France. Ellen Woodlock's recruitment drive had been a successful one and six Irish women entered the convent at Juilly at around the same time.

In Ireland, meanwhile, the Catholic Church was seizing the opportunity presented by new legislation to expand. The 1858 act 'to promote and regulate reformatory schools for juvenile offenders in Ireland' gave state support to institutions run by voluntary organisations for 'the better training of juvenile offenders'. Within a year six reformatories had opened, five of which were run

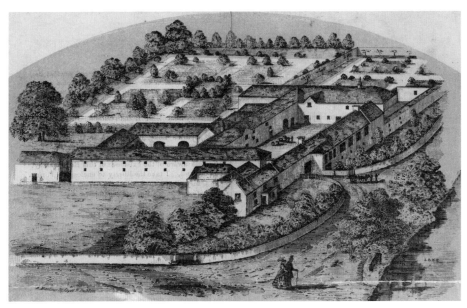

'Ulster Reformatory School for Catholic Girls, Monaghan' – originally Spark's Lake brewery, purchased for the St Louis nuns by Charles Bianconi. (St Louis Convent archive, Monaghan)

by Catholic groups and for the exclusive incarceration of Catholic children. In late 1858 a small but influential group began to plan for such an institution in Monaghan. John Lentaigne, the inspector of prisons, Mrs Lloyd, the mother of Lady Rossmore and also a convert, Ellen Woodlock, whose family owned the woollen mills at Blarney, and the bishop of Clogher decided to open a reformatory in Monaghan. Ellen Woodlock wrote that 'the bishop, Mrs Lloyd and Mr Lentaigne request a well-bred, well-educated French sister' for the task. The bishop wrote to the abbé in France to ask that a foundation of the St Louis order be established in Monaghan. Three sisters, Genevieve, Clare and Clement, arrived there on 6 January 1859 after an eventful journey from France, with very little money and an expectation that a house awaited them. There was no house and, after some nights spent in a hotel, they moved into a small, unfurnished house.

They survived for some time by teaching local children, until they were rescued by Charles Bianconi, who purchased an old brewery at Spark's Lake. The sisters moved into the brewery and received their first reformatory child on 14 October 1859. Ellen Brown was an eleven-year-old girl from Belfast who had seven convictions prior to her reformatory sentence. Genevieve Beale wrote of her that she 'presented a pale and emaciated appearance, from the habitual use of strong liquors, during the short periods when in the enjoyment of liberty, and owing to the rigours of a refractory cell, while undergoing punishment in gaol'.

DIETARY.

BREAKFAST.

Stirabout made with Indian Meal and Oatmeal, 1 pint of Milk.
Sunday :—From 8 to 12 oz. Bread, 1 pint of Cocoa.

DINNER.

Sunday and Thursday :—Beef and Vegetables, 1½ lbs. of Potatoes.
Monday, Wednesday, and Friday :—From 8 to 12 oz. of Bread,
1 pint of Soup.
Tuesday and Thursday :—1⅓ lbs. Potatoes, 1 pint of Milk.

SUPPER.

Daily :—8 oz. of Bread, 1 pint of Cocoa.

TIME TABLE.

CLASS OF HONOUR.—SIXTEEN GIRLS.

6 a.m.—Rise, wash, make beds.
6¼ „ —Family prayer.
7 „ —Household duties (a certain number of girls take lessons
in crotchet work, marking, &c.).
9 „ —Breakfast.
9½ „ —Recreation.
10 „ —Sewing class (a certain number go to the laundry and
kitchen).
3 p.m.—Dinner.
3½ „ —Out-door exercise and gardening, when the weather
permits.
5 „ —Occupied in school-room for three hours, learning cate-
chism, sacred history, reading, writing, arithmetic,
rudiments of geography, grammar, &c.
8 „ —Supper.
8½ „ —Family prayer.
9 „ —To bed.

*The daily timetable for the reformatories usually included six hours of work and three
of instruction. Some children were refused admission to the schools, especially the boys' schools, if
it was considered that they were too ill to work.*

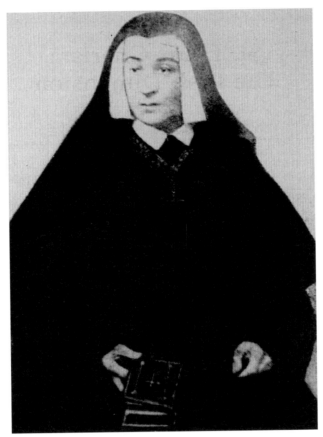

Sr Genevieve, the foundress of the Monaghan school, was a Catholic convert, born Priscilla Beale to Protestant, possibly Quaker, parents in London in 1822. (St Louis Convent archive, Monaghan).

By 1862 the inspector of reformatories was writing that the Monaghan school was receiving 'some of the most vicious and refractory girls' he had ever seen. These included girls who were rejected by other reformatories, such as prostitutes or those suffering from venereal diseases, and girls whose behaviour meant that other schools, particularly High Park in Dublin, could not cope with them. By 1865 the school had 39 inmates. The inspector said of Genevieve Beale that:

> Were it not for the manager's [Sr Beale's] indomitable perseverance in her mission, and her courage in accepting the transfer from High Park of the worst class of Dublin girls, eight at least would have been thrown upon the world and into utter depravity. There are none so wicked, so violent—so, to all human judgement, lost—as to be beyond the scope of her zeal and sympathy.

When the representatives of a government commission visited Spark's Lake in January 1883 they were told that, in its early years, such was the violence of some of the girls to each other and to themselves that strait waistcoats were provided and sometimes used.

When the Monaghan school opened, it described itself as being the only reformatory for Catholic girls in the north and west of Ireland. This situation would not change until 1864, when Connacht's only reformatory opened. On 7 December 1863 Mary Burke, the superior of the Mercy convent in Ballinasloe, wrote to the chief secretary, Robert Peel, that she had been preparing a building in the town for the reception of female juvenile offenders. She was acting under the direction of her bishop, Dr Derry. The inspector, whose job it was to recommend the building and the manager to the chief secretary, found a well-fitted-out building and a manager who was 'fully prepared to receive twelve children, and has the complete school uniform, with beds, bedding and bed clothing' when he visited. The new school received its first girl, Margaret Seery, in March 1864. Margaret was ten years old. She had been born in the workhouse and was described by the inspector as an 'inveterate thief' who had been trained to steal by her mother. She was arrested in Sligo with a woman, probably her mother, and found guilty of stealing a purse containing five shillings. She was given a sentence of one calendar month in Sligo gaol and five years in the new reformatory. Margaret found herself with few companions in her new home. Despite her preparations, Mary Burke's school was undersubscribed, so that by 1866 there were only nine inmates.

The great test of the reformatory system was that the children who were sent to the schools would leave them as honest and industrious individuals who were sufficiently trained to become self-supporting. 'Disposal of the inmates' was a challenge for all of the reformatory managers, and the inspector's office in Dublin Castle requested that they keep a record of those who were released for three years after they had left the institutions. Both Mary Burke and Genevieve Beale tried to find work for the girls when they left. In 1862 Genevieve Beale wrote that 'the future of our poor children is a source of increasing anxiety to us'. Mary Burke could tell the inspector in 1873 that, of the five girls discharged in the previous year, one remained in the school until a position was found for her in Ballinasloe, one had gone to her brother in New York, one was 'keeping house for her father', and two were 'giving perfect satisfaction' as general servants. Where it was felt that the girls would relapse into crime, or if their parents were criminal, great efforts were made to remove them from their former associates. In 1865 the inspector of reformatories reported what had happened in Monaghan when two girls—cousins—were about to be released from the school:

Their relatives, a gang of wandering tinkers, had been prowling about the reformatory, and were driven off by the constabulary. They went away, declaring their intention of returning on the day of the girls' discharge . . . A steamer was to sail from Londonderry three days before the expected day of discharge. [The manager] telegraphed me to obtain a pardon from the chief secretary at once . . . and three days before the day of discharge the two girls were sailing for New York.

The mother and grandmother of one of the girls were in convict prisons, and the father and brother of the other girl were in a prison and a reformatory. Genevieve Beale did not always succeed in removing the girls; two others were taken by their mothers at the expiration of their sentences in Monaghan 'to live upon the wages of their sin, although the money for their passage and outfit, and honest employment in Canada, were secured for them'.

For some of the discharged girls, their passage to North America would prove eventful. 'A.M.' emigrated to New York and was married 'immediately after landing' to one of the ship's crew. 'M.B.' received a proposal of marriage from the mate of the vessel in which she sailed to Boston, which she declined. 'C.T.' arrived at Monaghan a 'depraved and immoral girl' who had absconded from High Park and was the recipient of a similar proposal from a fellow passenger, a commercial traveller, en route to New York. She refused him, on finding that he was 'not religious'.

By the time that Bridget Carroll arrived in Monaghan, many changes had occurred in both the school that she was leaving and the one to which she was sent. Ballinasloe had never reached its capacity of inmates, although its numbers were boosted for a time by the transfer of refractory children from industrial schools. In 1883 Mary Burke applied for recertification of the reformatory as an industrial school. Her application was granted, and she remained the manager until 1894. When the representatives of the Reformatories and Industrial Schools Commission visited Spark's Lake four months before Bridget's arrival, they noted a 'general improvement in character of the committed children'. Genevieve Beale had died at the age of 56 in 1878. The school that she had founded closed in 1903. Bridget Carroll remained in Monaghan until October 1884. She emigrated to New York and in the two years after her discharge was reported to be 'doing well'.

Chapter Nine

Casement's 'Black diaries': Closed books reopened

Angus Mitchell

Roger Casement (1864-1916), humanitarian and Irish revolutionary, was put on trial at the end of June 1916 on a charge of high treason against the British Crown which he had served as a conscientious consul in both Africa (1895-1904) and South America (1906-13), until his resignation from the Foreign Office in the summer of 1913 when he began to devote his energies to the cause of Irish freedom. At the end of October 1914 British intelligence services got wind of Casement's efforts to bring about a German-Irish alliance and despite efforts to undermine his activities, it was not until April 1916 that he was eventually arrested on Banna Strand, County Kerry, just hours before the outbreak of the Easter Rising.

On the fourth and last day of his trial, in an exchange in court between the Attorney-General, Sir F.E. Smith—leading the prosecution—and the chief justice, reference was made for the first time to 'Casement's diary'. When rumours began to percolate among newspapers, politicians, ambassadors and gentlemen's clubs in July 1916 about Roger Casement's 'sexual degeneracy' those who had known him most closely found it hardest to believe. But in that dark apocalyptic summer of 1916 it was doubtless reconciled in the minds of most, that if a man was capable of co-operating with Germany—and had himself admitted to treason—then he was capable of anything.

In the month between his trial and execution, as the battle of the Somme raged on the Western Front, no less than six petitions were raised urging the government to grant a reprieve. But on 18 July a cabinet memorandum made reference, for the first time, to the 'Black Diaries'. It alleged that the documents clearly showed that Casement 'had for years been addicted to the grossest sodomitical practices'. Material circulated at the highest government level in both Britain and the United States, wholly undermining the campaign for clemency and successfully preventing Casement attaining martyrdom. Early in the morning of 3 August 1916 Roger Casement was hanged.

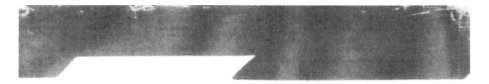

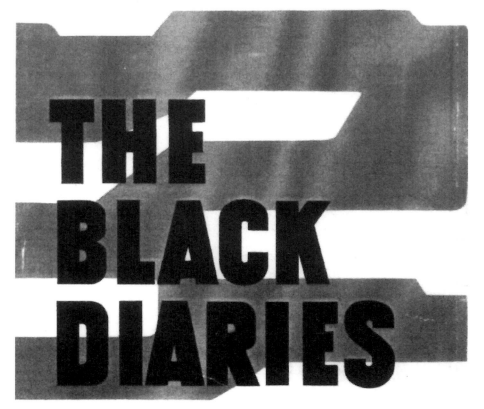

The Black Diaries by Peter Singleton-Gates and Maurice Girodias.

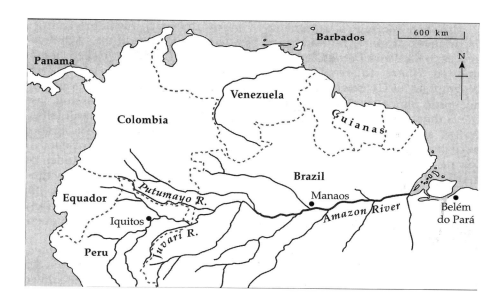

In 1959 the veil of secrecy over the contents of the 'Black Diaries' was finally lifted with their lavish publication in Paris, outside the jurisdiction of the British Crown, by the Fleet Street newspaperman, Peter Singleton-Gates and the publisher of censored material, Maurice Girodias. In his foreword to the book, Singleton-Gates related how:

> In May 1922 a person of some authority in London presented me with a bundle of documents, with the comment that if ever I had time I might find in them the basis for a book of unusual interest. The donor had no ulterior motive for wishing such a book published: his gift was no more than a kind gesture to a journalist and writer.

In the mid–1990s the declassification of flies relating to Casement revealed that Singleton-Gates had acted as a 'front' for the head of Special Branch, Sir Basil Thomson, the man credited with discovering the Black Diaries. It was Thomson who handed Singleton-Gates the typescripts of the Black Diaries following his dismissal from New Scotland Yard after a breach of public decency laws.

But at the time the act of publishing the Black Diaries, as they were now christened, seemed to endorse the genuineness of the documents. From 10 August 1959 the Home Secretary permitted historical researchers to see manuscript material which generally corresponded with Singleton-Gates's faulty published text. Despite considerable interest in the British and Irish press the only effort at anything near a scholarly analysis was a short essay by an Irish academic, Roger

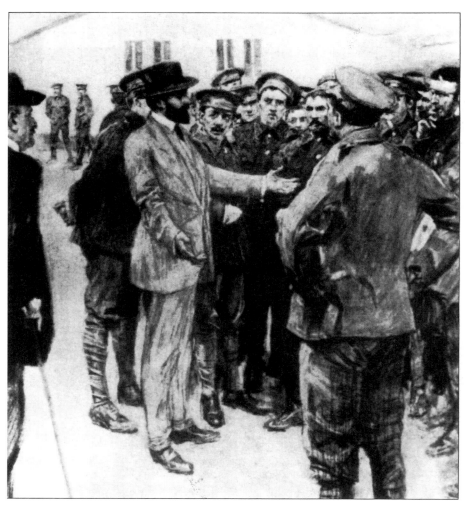

In his German Diaries, Casement recorded his efforts to recruit an Irish Brigade from amongst captured prisoners-of-war, depicted here in a painting by W. Hatherell. (Mansell Collection).

McHugh who cast doubt on the serious discrepancies between the diaries held in the Public Record Office (now the National Archives of the United Kingdom) and eyewitness accounts of material exhibited in 1916 as Casement's diary. He showed suspicious internal discrepancies and contradictions. He demonstrated how the chronology of the diary campaign, establishing their alleged discovery, was part of a wartime propagandist intelligence initiative against Casement launched well before his arrest. Finally, he analysed how official accounts of the provenance of the Black Diaries were mutually contradictory.

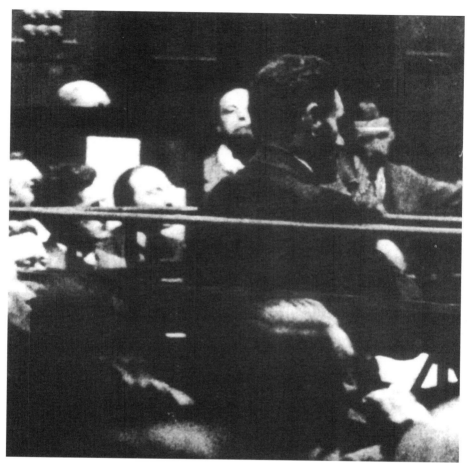

Casement in the dock, 16 May 1916.

Although McHugh's arguments were never properly refuted, once access to the Black Diaries had been granted, there followed several biographies of Casement. Each one accepted almost without question the authenticity of the Black Diaries. As the social taboos about homosexuality began to break down following the sexual revolution of the sixties, Casement's 'treason' and 'homosexuality' were attractive characteristics for biographers and publishers anxious to sell books.

Casement's life was interpreted in terms of paradoxes—he was seen as a 'fragmented and elusive' character, but nevertheless a man capable of protecting native peoples on one hand whilst quietly 'perverting' them to satisfy his mounting sexual libido. His sexuality mirrored his treason and his ambivalent and contradictory character—extending from 'emotional deprivation, religious uncertainties, the duality of his political commitments'—was bound up with his 'sexual perversion' and homosexuality. No longer the 'sexual degenerate', Casement was now transformed into the 'gay traitor'. But in no way do the Black Diaries serve the LGBT community or merit a place in twentieth-century homosexual literature. Whoever wrote the diaries portrayed homosexuality as a sickness and perversion and crime for which a person should suffer guilt, repression, fantasy, hatred and most of all, alienation and loneliness. These are not the confessions of a Jean Genet or Tennessee Williams, W.H. Auden or Oscar Moore. Rather than sympathising with the struggle of the homosexual conscience they are clearly homophobic documents.

Brian Inglis's *Roger Casement* (1973) placed his subject in the context of other well-known homosexuals—André Gide. Marcel Proust, Oscar Wilde. His argument against the forgery theory was brief but adamant:

> Nevertheless the case against the forgery theory remains unshaken. No person or persons, in their right mind, would have gone to so much trouble and expense to damn a traitor when a single diary would have sufficed. To ask the forger to fake the other two diaries and the cash register (and if one were forged, all of them were) would have been simply to ask for detection, because a single mistake in any of them would have destroyed the whole ugly enterprise. Besides, where could the money have been found? Government servants may sometimes be unscrupulous, but they are always tight-fisted .

Following the release of the Black Diaries in March 1994 and over 170 previously closed Casement files in October 1995 (now available to readers at NAUK) the whole matter of 'Casement's diaries' was effectively deemed to be history.

The Black Diaries consist of five hard-back books of varying size. The first, known as the Army Book—a small field service notebook—is an apparently innocuous document with the first entry referring to the death of Queen Victoria and brief entries between 6 and 13 February 1902 and short accounts of Casement's movements on 20 and 21 July 1902 when he was travelling in the Belgian Congo. It holds no obvious sexual references and is filled with a few abstract notes about distances and railway times, transcriptions from foreign newspapers and two rough sketch maps.

The first 'Black Diary' is a small Letts's Pocket Diary & Almanac—covering the months of Casement's investigation into the Congo from 14 February 1903 to 8 January 1904 with a few notes added on at the beginning and end. The diary records sexual acts in London, Congo, Madeira, Canary Islands and Sierra Leone, mainly with native boys.

The next is a Dollard's 1910 Office Diary, most of which coincides with Casement's first voyage to the Amazon at the end of July 1910 and continues uninterrupted until the end of the year. Sex or sexual fantasies occur in Rio de Janeiro, São Paulo, Mar del Plata, London, Belfast, Dublin and with most frequency up the Amazon at Belém do Pará, Manaos, Iquitos and in the Putumayo.

The 1911 Letts's Desk Diary—never published and the most explicit and pornographic in content—follows on directly from the last entry for 31 December in the 1910 Dollard's Diary. After day-by-day entries for the first eighteen days of January, as Casement spent New Year in Paris before returning to London after his first Amazon voyage there is a rough sketch (unidentified) covering a page in February, and a very untypical signature 'Sir Roger Casement CMG' opposite May, the month Casement received news of his knighthood. After that the diary is blank until 13 August when the entries resume and detail the movements that coincide with his second voyage up the Amazon to Iquitos and into the Brazilian-Peruvian frontier region of the river Javari. During this journey the sexual references are almost of daily occurrence and of the most plainly explicit nature. Long, cryptic entries of fantasy mix with nights of exceptional sexual athletics and endless descriptions of cruising along the waterfronts of Belém do Pará, Manaos and Iquitos. The most explicit entry takes place on Sunday 1 October, the start of the pheasant shooting season in England. By this account the diarist did little on this journey except fantasise and seek out willing sexual partners or seduce underage boys at every opportunity. After a short stay in Iquitos and an expedition to try and arrest some of the fugitive slave-drivers, the document details the return down the Amazon to Belém do Pará and then north to Barbados. At the end are a couple of pages of figures detailing expenditure during the voyage.

The last diary, known as the 'Cash ledger', is a record of daily accounts written in a blank hard-back cash book. It briefly records 'expenditure' for February and March 1910 and then begins a day-by-day account of financial out-goings for 1911 from 1 January to 31 October. At the end there are a few more brief entries about 1910. A number of sexual references look as if they have been interpolated into the text.

The physical characteristics of the Black Diaries vary significantly from the journal that Casement kept during his 1910 Amazon voyage (both manuscript and typescript versions are held by the National Library of Ireland) and whose authenticity has never been doubted. This document is written on 128 unbound loose leaves of lined, double-sided foolscap and covers the period from 23 September to 6 December 1910, the seventy-five days that Casement spent travelling through the Putumayo and his return to and departure from

Iquitos. It is the document that is variously referred to as the 'white diary' or 'the cleaned-up version', since it does not contain any sexual acts or fantasies. For the purposes of clear identification in this argument it is referred to as the Putumayo Journal.

Other important documents are Casement's German diaries (held in the National Library of Ireland). Beginning on 7 November 1914, they record his efforts to recruit an Irish Brigade from amongst captured prisoners-of-war in Germany. They throw revealing light on how conscientious Casement was about his diaries and on the form such journals or diaries took. Before leaving Munich at the end of March 1916 Casement entrusted to his German solicitor, Charles Curry, 'all he possessed in this world, his personal effects and writings and left various instructions chiefly regarding his diaries and their publication upon the close of war'. From looking at the nature and provenance of the various diaries it becomes clear that Casement conscientiously kept diaries or journals during large parts of his life and that these were most detailed during the more momentous occasions, either during his humanitarian investigations or his last adventure as a leader of the 1916 Rising. It also seems probable that a large number of these personal notes fell into the hands of British Intelligence when Casement's London rooms were raided, and his possessions seized sometime during the eighteen-month period between the realisation by British Intelligence that Casement was a dangerous traitor to the moment of his arrest in April 1916.

Through constructing a narrative of Casement's 1910 Amazon voyage from undisputed documentation, whether journals, fragmentary entries or letters, it is possible to compare it with the narrative of his trip as told in the 1910 Black Diary. It becomes clear that the Black Diary is riddled with inaccuracies and inconsistencies that describe events in a completely different way. There is no information contained in parallel entries of the Black Diary that could not have been copied from the Putumayo Journal. Besides sexual references, the only information contained in the Black Diary and not included in the Putumayo Journal regarded general matters such as water levels, the climate and descriptions of flora and fauna. It also becomes impossible to contend, therefore, that Casement used a shortened Black Diary to write subsequently his Putumayo Journal.

Those who wish to continue believing in the genuineness of the Black Diaries should ask themselves why Casement would have kept such an incriminating document about his person when he realised that in South America his every step was being watched and he was moving through an atmosphere of fear, suspicion and death? Indeed, why whould he leave such personally-damaging material behind him when he defected to Germany at the start of the war?

The figure of Roger Casement who emerges from the Putumayo Journal is so different in general attitude and moral values from the Casement portrayed by the Black Diaries as to be totally irreconcilable.

The Putumayo Journal, fragmentary diary entries and Foreign Office dispatches are all written in Casement's clear and succinct English prose. Throughout he is lucid, emotional, direct, structured and thoughtful. It is filled with intelligent comments by a man with a highly active, inquiring mind and touches on a number of different subjects—including botany, ethnology, anthropology, history, politics, race and religion—whilst keeping its eye firmly on the matter in hand: compiling a case against perpetrators of atrocities in the wild rubber trade. It is arguably the most important surviving document Casement wrote and shows what a remarkably controlled and clear mind he possessed even when he was physically suffering and under enormous danger.

The Black Diaries by contrast have been written to mystify, befuddle, confuse and conceal. More often than not they are utterly misleading in their meaning. Far from appearing as a serious-minded figure, they portray Casement as a perverter of the innocent, a corrupter and indecent fantasist. The language is charged with innuendo and exaggeration. The genuine phraseology Casement adopts to describe the 'noble savage' as a handsome, strong and innocent human being has been twisted to give it an ambiguous sexual connotation. Sense has been confused, truth obscured. Characters have been extracted from their genuine context and given new roles as sexual partners or objects of fantasy. Recently, using detailed computerised analysis of key-words and expressions, Eoin Ó Máille and Michael Payne have shown that the linguistic finger-print in Casement's undisputed writings is completely at odds with the linguistic finger-print of the Black Diaries.

Casement's recent biographers have explained the existence of these two parallel diaries in terms of a sex diary and a 'cleaned up version'—a 'black' and a 'white' diary—as if Casement was a Jekyll and Hyde character. The argument can appear convincing if it is put in the context of the fact that for most of this century, certainly during Casement's lifetime, homosexuality was driven underground, and homosexuals until recently were forced to lead double lives. But such an argument fails to take into account the incredibly small and hostile world in which Casement moved in South America and the fact that his every move, whilst investigating in one of the most wild, dangerous frontier regions of the world was being watched by enemies who wished him dead.

Analysed as texts, once Casement's undisputed narrative is compared to corresponding Black Diary entries it becomes impossible to believe in the authenticity of both. The genuineness of the diaries has always depended upon the argument that they were factually fool-proof. The most blatant inconsistency concerns Casement's eyes. On re-entering tropical climes Casement started to suffer a desperate eye infection. The eye problem followed him from Iquitos to La Chorrera, the capital of the Putumayo district and the base from which Casement began his investigations. His sick eyes dogged him constantly for the next month and the Putumayo Journal has a string of references to his eyes until the night of 12 October when the problem reached a climax and Casement was forced to bandage both eyes when he went to bed. He had effectively realised his worst nightmare and gone blind in the depths of the Amazon forest.

Despite over fifteen separate mentions of his eyes between 11 August and 12 October in the Putumayo Journal the first mention in the Black Diary is on 10 October—fully two months after Casement had first mentioned the problem and just two days before both his eyes broke down and he was rendered temporarily blind. Casement's eye infection was so bad that it forced him to use pencil; it also forced him to be as economic with his writing as possible and to avoid unnecessary strain. Why then is it supposed he was keeping two separate journals repeating the same information? A harder question to answer is why at the very moment when his eyes were at their worst and clearly affecting his script in the Putumayo Journal is the Black Diary entry for 12 October written in small and deliberate well-formed black ink?

According to the Black Diary and Casement's most recent biographers, on arriving at Iquitos on 31 August he took up residence at the Hotel Cosmopolite. Yet there is no record of this in the expense accounts Casement subsequently submitted to the Foreign Office. The claim is flatly contradicted by Casement's own reports to the Foreign Office that he stayed with the British vice consul David Cazes.

Another point that makes little sense is an uncharacteristically personal comment made by Casement about his sexuality on 29 September, after he had witnessed, in the company of the perpetrators of atrocities, his first Indian dance at the rubber station of Occidente:

> I swear to God, I'd hang every one of the band of wretches with my own hands if I had the power, and do it with the greatest pleasure. I have never shot game with any pleasure, have indeed abandoned all shooting for that reason, that I dislike the thought of taking life. I have never given life to anyone myself, and my celibacy makes me frugal of human life, but I'd shoot or exterminate these infamous scoundrels more gladly than I should shoot a crocodile or kill a snake.

Exactly why Casement should have made such a direct statement about his celibacy whilst keeping a parallel sex diary is a contradiction which has yet to be explained by those who still find it possible to believe in both 'black' and 'white' diaries. There is not a single witness to Casement's alleged sexual antics on the Amazon as detailed by the 1910 and 1911 Black Diaries and certainly South America was the main theatre for his alleged sexual degeneracy if the documents are believed genuine. Moreover Casement's principal enemy on the Amazon, the Peruvian rubber baron, Julio Cesar Arana, knew all about Casement's 'secret' activities, such as recruiting labour for the Madeira-Mamore railway and trying to organise an anti-Aranista party during his second voyage to Iquitos in 1911. In December 1911, when Casement made a hasty exit from Iquitos, the local newspapers were accusing him of being a 'British spy' and 'secret agent', but all such suggestions are edited out of the Black Diary. Eighty years on these documents continue to confuse and confound.

How and why did British intelligence go to such complicated lengths to forge the Black Diaries? The strategy had both short-term and long-term objectives. The short-term aim was to secure Casement's execution. They were an effective way to mislead his powerful lobby of supporters and officially to defame Sir Roger Casement—the humanitarian hero, knighted in 1911 for his epic journeys in defence of rainforest communities on behalf of the British Crown. They are an example of a type of ruthless intellectual sabotage, which the British excel at when it is a matter of defeating the enemy. The Black Diaries were first rumoured in the aftermath of 1916 and, given the nature of Casement's self-proclaimed treason, they were an exceptional weapon deployed to assassinate the character of an exceptional enemy.

The process of forging the documents was comparatively easy although it undoubtedly required great expertise in its execution. When British intelligence moved in on Casement at the end of 1914, among his confiscated papers they found genuine diaries and journals detailing his journeys into the Congo and Putumayo. Using this material they were able, without too much difficulty, to construct the Black Diaries with experiences, phraseology and impressions cannibalised from genuine writings. On the surface these documents appeared to be factually fool-proof and contained a host of references and indications to give the appearance of being genuine documents. Certainly the forging of the handwriting was carried out with great skill, although since there is no evidence that the Black Diaries held in the Public Records Office were described by anyone in 1916, it is probable that the forger had several years to perfect their look. Though the formation of letters and the style of the writing is often hard to distinguish from genuine material, it ultimately fails the test of authenticity for its total lack of fluency. All Casement's writings, whether notes, letters or journals contain a fluency of script—as if Casement was working under enormous pressure and at great speed. The Black Diaries completely lack this. The words seem to stutter out onto the page—they are deliberate and contrived.

The rumours of Casement's 'sexual degeneracy' that were circulated before and after his trial in 1916 confused almost everyone. Casement's powerful lobby of supporters retreated into silence. Casement's martyrdom was prevented and the clemency appeals thwarted. His Irish supporters were in retreat, devastated by the execution of the leaders of the Easter Rising. All were fearful of speaking out in defence of a man whose treason was so clear, at a time when each day tens of thousands of British volunteers were being slaughtered on the front-line of the Somme. For the rest of this century the Black Diaries became the means by which Casement's 'treason' was explained and rationalised in public.

There was however a secondary motive for forging the Black Diaries that becomes clear once the documents are analysed outside the confines of the Anglo-Irish conflict and the First World War. His investigations into atrocities in both the Congo and Amazon are unique, officially-sanctioned sources in understanding the horror that underlay wild rubber extraction from tropical forests. In these investigations Casement collected the statements and oral testimonies that helped build a factual case supporting the historical heart of darkness that lay in the shadowy soul of European imperialism and the white man's vision of civilisation. Although the Black Diaries make impressionistic references to the horror, they cleverly scale the horror down, Casement emerges as the 'degenerate' rather than the imperial systems he was investigating. It is no coincidence that the Black Diaries coincide with Casement's main humanitarian investigations into rubber atrocities in both Africa and South America, and most specifically with the Putumayo atrocities where British financial influence was most active and direct.

Chapter Ten

Roger Casement and the history question

Angus Mitchell

Irrespective of the question of their authenticity, it is now universally agreed that the Black Diaries were integral to a smear campaign conjured up in 1916 to railroad Roger Casement to the gallows and deny him the moral high ground that helped to justify the Irish rebellion. *One bold deed of open treason: The Berlin diary of Roger Casement 1914–1916* (2016) becomes my third edited volume in the retrieval of the Casement archive. This project began back in 1997 with the publication of *The Amazon journal of Roger Casement* and was followed by *Sir Roger Casement's heart of darkness* (2003). These initial two volumes enabled a deeper reading of the critical years 1910 and 1911. This third edition covers Casement's time in Germany following the outbreak of the First World War. Cumulatively, the volumes provide insight into one of the more complex and misunderstood Irish activists of the revolutionary generation and his internationalism. On another level, the texts facilitate a new way of analysing the Black Diaries' controversy.

In his Berlin diary, Casement divulges his deeper political intentions behind diary-writing. On his departure from Germany for Ireland in April 1916, he left clear and explicit instructions for the safekeeping of this document, despite the fact that it was intentionally self-incriminating and explained the logic behind his treason. In his own words, the reader is led into an entangled conspiracy against his former British Foreign Office colleagues. The narrative begins during the July crisis of 1914, with Casement arriving in New York (spied on from every side) to liaise and plot with the Irish Republican Brotherhood executive. His own credibility with other revolutionary leaders reaches a high point in the wake of the successful landing of guns at Howth and Kilcoole. In late October, after leaving the US, Casement passed through Christiania (Oslo) on his way to Berlin. By then he had become a high security risk and efforts were made by British secret services to have him 'knocked on the head'—in short, assassinated.

In Berlin, Casement entered into a long process of negotiations with different tentacles of Imperial Germany's wartime government. His journey through

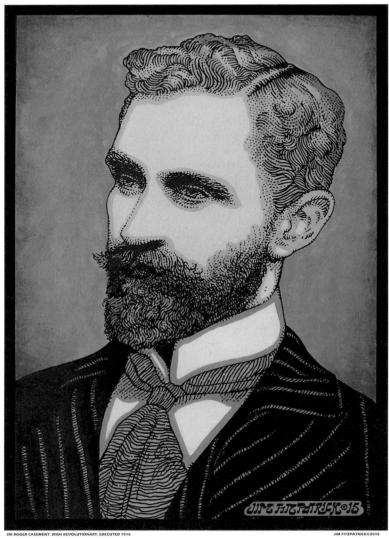

Sir Roger Casement, Irish revolutionary. Executed 1916. (Jim Fitzpatrick).

Belgium to the Western Front to meet senior officers in the German general staff is described. He details his subsequent conversation with the chancellor, Theobald von Bethmann Hollweg, and other senior politicians. His largely futile efforts to raise an Irish Brigade display deepening levels of frustration. The diary cuts out from late February 1915 to March 1916; then it revives as Casement prepares to leave Germany for Ireland to try and stop the rebellion or stand and die beside his comrades.

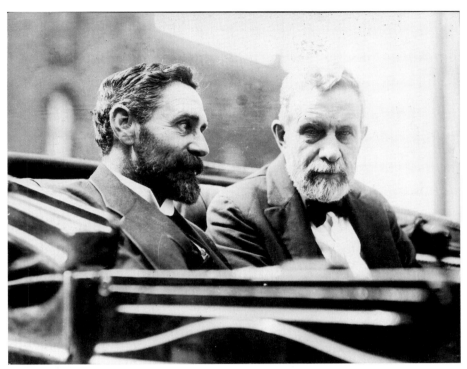

Casement with John Devoy, leader of Clan na Gael, in New York during the July crisis of 1914, where the Berlin diary narrative begins. (Villanova University).

Beyond what the diary tells us of Casement's 'treason', the narrative provides intriguing insight into the covert world of both British and German wartime intelligence agencies. His heated encounters with the German spymaster Rudolf Nadolny (grandfather of the acclaimed German novelist Sten Nadolny, author of *The discovery of slowness*) afford insight into the inner workings of the Prussian war machine. On another level, the deepening intrigue exposes further motives as to why the question of Casement's diaries persisted as an issue. In the course of his Berlin confession, Casement describes how he consciously forges extracts from his diary in a scheme to deceive the British Foreign Office. When lengthy excerpts from the Berlin diary were published in the US, Ireland and Germany during the signing and implementation of the Anglo-Irish treaty between November 1921 and February 1922, the spectre of the Black Diaries returned.

In a sense Casement *was* a 'gay martyr': the incitement of popular homophobia was intrinsic to ensuring his execution and denigrating his meaning among his national and international networks of support. Moreover, there are revealing links between his trial and the later negotiations of Irish independence.

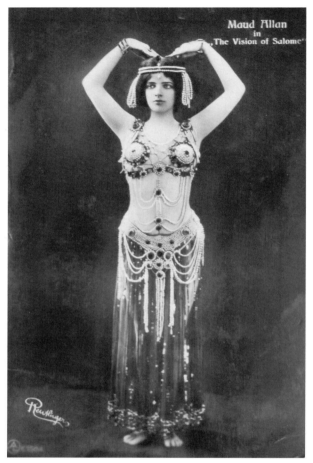

Maud Allan in The vision of Salome, a loose adaptation of the Oscar Wilde play.

Casement's prosecutor, Lord Birkenhead, and his defence solicitor, George Gavan Duffy, were both signatories of the Anglo-Irish Treaty. Authentication of the Black Diaries became part of the secret negotiation in the background to the treaty. Their endorsement was part of the secret history of the Irish independence struggle. Why else would Michael Collins have opened an official file series in 1922 labelled 'Alleged Casement Diaries'?

This set the Irish state down the road of a deeply ambivalent relationship with both the Black Diaries and Casement. On one side, there was a need to recognise the role that Casement played in the move towards and justification of rebellion and as a founding father of an independent Irish foreign policy. On the other side, accepting the authenticity of the Black Diaries was an

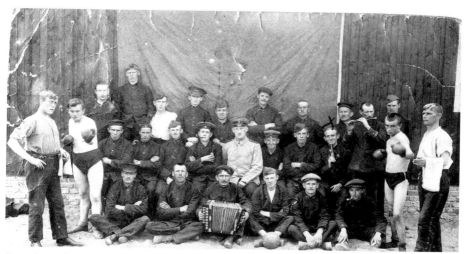

Recruits to Casement's Irish Brigade pictured in Germany – half of the total of 56 who joined up. His largely futile efforts to raise an Irish Brigade caused him deepening levels of frustration. (National Museum of Ireland)

undisclosed element in the Irish Free State deal. This unplayable hand would define the dispute over Casement's legacy in the Anglo-Irish history wars of the next century and culminating in this year of commemoration.

In England, the diaries helped in a different type of cultural construction, leading to the disremembering of Casement within British imperial history. After years of denial of their very existence, the Black Diaries passed in 1959 into the custody of the Public Record Office. Researchers seeking access were carefully vetted by the Home Office and required permission from the incumbent home secretary. On the return of Casement's remains to Ireland in 1965, a further understanding was agreed between London and Dublin that essentially closed down open discussion on the diaries' controversy for another 30 years.

During that period, public consensus regarding the veracity of the Black Diaries was built through the publication of a steady stream of psychological biographies that locked the Black Diaries into the heart of Casement's life. This intervention primed Casement to become a 'gay icon' as much as a national liberator. But messages remained mixed.

In the summer of 1994, on the release of the Black Diaries into the public domain, Professor Paul Bew wrote a controversial article in *History Ireland* arguing unequivocally for the authenticity of the diaries. A few months later, Professor Stephen Howe, reviewing Edward Said's *Orientalism* for the *New Statesman* (24 February 1995), commented that 'the diary was almost certainly forged by the British government to aid in railroading Casement to the gallows'.

Howe's comment hinted at a 'knowingness' or subjugated knowledge that has informed the view about Casement from within the historical academy. But in Howe's *Ireland and empire* (2000) Casement received passing mention, despite a deepening recognition amongst post-colonial theorists of the latter's damning critique of western imperialism. Tension and dissonance within élite academic circles were set to continue.

Publication of *The Amazon journal* in 1997 had drawn attention to the fact that there was much confusion over the relationship between 'Black' and 'White' diary narratives describing the same 75-day period during 1910 when Casement investigated the activities of a British-owned Peruvian rubber company. This opened the controversy to another kind of scrutiny that was scholarly and textual and not politically constrained and luridly sexual. *The Amazon journal* demonstrated how Casement was deconstructing the racist logic of empire. His incisive analysis exposed the gender-based violence supporting international venture capital. To a shocked metropolitan audience, he revealed the resource wars fought in the name of civilisation against peaceful, indigenous communities and their environments. The fact that the Black Diaries configured so precisely with his investigations into atrocities in the Congo Free State in 1903 and in the north-western Amazon in 1910 and 1911 was becoming their most revealing weakness.

It is now evident that the Black Diaries have enabled their own form of epistemological violence, whereby Casement's achievement as both a pioneer of human rights and a whistle-blower could be marginalised by accusing him of paedophilia. If the Black Diaries are to be placed centre stage to their biographical subject, then their author, even in today's terms, was not engaging with 'hospitable bodies' but was using his position in deeply exploitative power games. Revisionist efforts to try and turn the sexualised Casement into a kind of Proustian hero, or a gay role model, do not stand up to rigorous scrutiny of the texts. Besides the homophobic world in which they were conjured, the diaries are deeply racist. By manipulating meaning, they demean the authority of the investigator. Casement's cultural construct as an urbane and playful cosmopolitan queer has little to do with the encrypted distortions evident in the sexualised version of events.

Like other revolutionary leaders involved in 1916, Casement was acutely aware of his place in history and the centrality of the written word to that place. As a British civil servant, he was aware, too, of the role of the archive in the production of history. I have long argued that his most subversive act was to leave on the official record an indelible indictment of colonial power: a denunciation that western historiography is still reluctant to acknowledge. Heading towards his own violent end on the scaffold—with the role of sexuality in the demise of both Parnell and Wilde still in living memory—is it really probable that he would have so conveniently left the ingredients for the subversion of his pioneering investigations? In any interrogation of the Black Diaries, questions to do with motive and probability weigh heavily on the side of forgery.

At the Irish state commemoration at Banna Strand on 21 April 2016, the British ambassador to Ireland, Dominick Chilcott, when interviewed by Radio Kerry, claimed that Casement's 'memory was lost in the [British] national consciousness'. Part of the process for that disremembering has been accomplished through the presence of the Black Diaries. Another motive for the forgery was to cover up a huge crime against humanity: a destruction of communities and environment that stretches from the upper Congo to the north-west Amazon to the destitute fringes of Connemara. Millions of dead souls—souls without history—haunt the shadows of Casement's tragedy. In his challenge to the imperial order, Casement blew the whistle on this catastrophe, and his engagement with revolutionary politics was a way by which he articulated his deepest sense of outrage against the system.

Britain's example of disremembering operates in direct opposition to what the theologian Johann Metz has described as the need to collectively connect with 'dangerous memories'. Casement is one such memory. Engaging with his life and death demands that we critically confront the victims and suffering created by the complacent structures of western power. His life opens up challenging perspectives on history and remembrance and their continuing interaction.

Surely if Ireland is now 'mature' enough to welcome the British monarch into its midst, then the UK's National Archive, without pageantry, can reattribute the Black Diaries. Thereby acts of interpretative violence can cease and Casement can be accepted as a rebel with a cause, whose memory should hold historic value and respect on both sides of the Irish Sea and beyond.

Chapter Eleven

Dancing, depravity and all that jazz: The Public Dance Halls Act of 1935

Jim Smyth

Aprotracted war of independence and a bitter civil war left the new Irish Free State with economic and social problems of enormous proportions - the economy and infrastructure were ravaged; unemployment and ill-health were endemic, and the wounds of the civil war were far from healed. But the agenda of perhaps the most powerful organised force in the country - the Catholic Church - was noticeably different.

In their Lenten pastorals of 1924 the Catholic bishops made their preoccupations unmistakably clear: 'The Irish bishops in their Lenten pastorals refer to the existence of many abuses. Chief among these may be mentioned women's fashions, immodest dress, indecent dancing, theatrical performances and cinema exhibitions, evil literature, drink, strikes and lock-outs'. Among this litany of putative abuses, one obsession remained constant and central for the next decade: the dangers attributed to the morals of the young posed by unlicensed dance halls and unsupervised dancing of any sort. This popular rural pastime became a classic terrain of fantasy projection and pseudo-knowledge, involving a potent brew of alleged sources of evil and degradation: cars, darkness, jazz music and the prospect of illicit and unsupervised dalliance between the sexes. Just as the advent of the railways was treated with horror by a section of Victorian England, and the bicycle was condemned by *The Times* in 1898 as adding an ominous dimension of mobility to the 'organised terrorism of the streets', the motor car was seen as an instrument of seduction in the hands of unscrupulous males. Cardinal Joseph MacRory in his pastoral letter of 1931 stressed the danger of too much mobility: 'Even the present travelling facilities make a difference. By bicycle, motor car and bus, boys and girls can now travel great distances to dances, with the result that a dance in the quietest country parish may now be attended by unsuitables from a distance'.

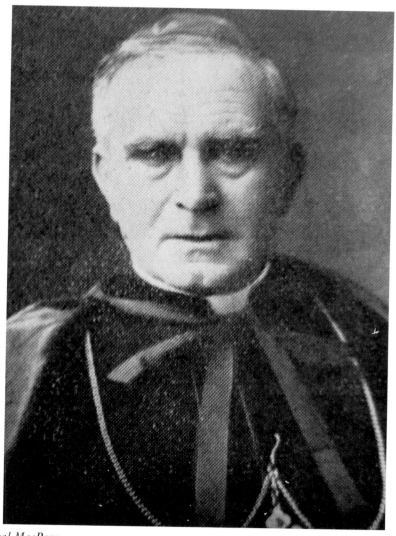

Cardinal MacRory.

The clergy were not against dancing in principle, as long as the dances were 'Irish' (a category confined, of course, to the modest ceilí dances and not the wilder and less restrained set dances) and the supervision was close. MacRory's predecessor Cardinal Michael Logue had set the tone in his pastoral of 1924:

> It is no small commendation of Irish dances that they cannot be danced for long hours. That, however, is not their chief merit. And while it is not part of our business to condemn any decent dance, Irish dances are not to be put

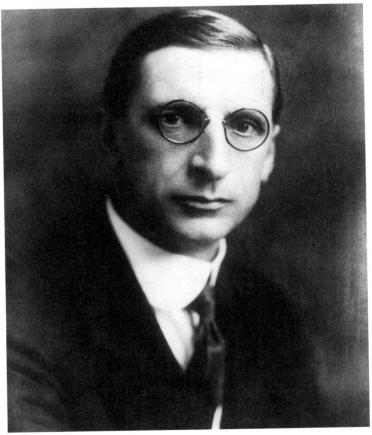

Eamonn de Valera gave his blessing to the anti-jazz campaign.

out of the place that is their due in any educational establishment under our care. They may not be the fashion in London and Paris. They should be the fashion in Ireland. Irish dances do not make degenerates.

During the latter half of the twenties, the demands of the bishops for legislation on personal morality became more vocal, an implicit admission that the church was unable to stem the rising tide of immorality which they claimed had engulfed the Free State after 1922. The focus of the campaign for legislative change was the amendment of the Criminal Law Amendment Acts of 1880 and 1885 (Stead's Act) which were originally enacted to combat juvenile prostitution, protect minors and make brothel keeping an offence. The fact that one in six houses in London was a brothel during that period may have had something to do with the passing of this Act. The government response was the Carrigan Committee (called after its

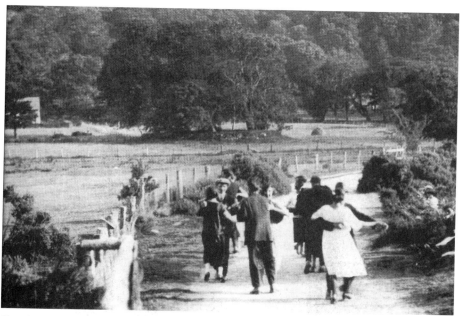

Dancing on the road at Glendalough Co. Wicklow in the late 1920s.

chairman, the senior barrister William Carrigan) which reported in 1931, having heard a large number of witnesses in private. None of this evidence was published in the press and the final report was never published. The committee interpreted its brief as nothing less than an inquiry into the moral state of the country:

> Under the terms of our reference we had to consider the secular aspect of social morality which is, the concern of the state to conserve and safeguard for the protection and well-being of its citizens. We looked upon it as our duty in the first place to collect sufficient information from such authentic sources as would enable us to determine whether the standard of social morality is at present exposed to evils, which the existing laws of the Saorstat for the suppression and prevention of public vice, are inadequate to check, and, should they be in our opinion inadequate, to consider how best they can be made effectual.

The report made it clear from the start that its conclusions were unanimous and that this unanimity even stretched to those giving evidence before the committee:

> No witness appearing before us has dissented from the view expressed by nearly every witness that the moral condition of the country has become

gravely menaced by modern abuses, widespread and pernicious in their consequences, which cannot be counteracted unless the laws of the state are revised and consistently enforced so as to combat them.

The committee, having established the dreadful moral state of the country, then proceeded to uncover the causes. The conclusion arrived at was that illegitimacy was in large measure to blame: 'Illegitimacy must be regarded as one of the principal causes of the species of crime and vice of which the state takes cognisance in the branch of penal and preventative legislation which we were appointed to examine'.

Although the report did not spell it out, the implication was clear. Young unmarried mothers were forced into prostitution because of their fallen state, and, indeed, could constitute an occasion of sin for others during confinement in Poor Law institutions: 'it is an objectionable fact that unmarried mothers of first-born children cannot be maintained apart from other inmates (the decent poor and sick)'. The report then moves on to the reasons for the alleged rise in illegitimacy and lays the blame clearly at the door of the dance halls:

> The testimony of all witnesses, clerical, lay and official, is striking in its unanimity that degeneration in the standard of social conduct has taken place in recent years. It is to be attributed primarily to the loss of parental control and responsibility during a period of general upheaval, which has not been recovered since the revival of settled conditions. This is due largely to the introduction of new phases of popular amusement, which being carried out in the Saorstát in the absence of supervision, and of the restrictions found necessary and enforced by law in other countries, are the occasions of many abuses baneful in their effect upon the community generally and are the cause of the ruin of hundreds of young girls, of whom many are found in the streets of London, Liverpool and other cities and towns in England. The 'commercialised' dance halls, picture houses of sorts, and the opportunities afforded by the misuse of motor cars for luring girls, are the chief causes alleged for the present looseness of morals.

Social conditions were hardly conducive to the standards of morality demanded by the clergy. The census of 1926 found that 800,000 people were living in overcrowded conditions – defined as more than two to a room – more than 25% of the population. Infant mortality among the Dublin working classes was 25.6 per 1,000 births as compared to 7.7 per 1,000 among the middle classes. The illegitimacy rate was 30.7 per 1,000 births for the country as a whole, although this figure showed considerable regional variations. The fact that 80% of all males between the ages of 25 and 30 were unmarried, as were 62% of all females in the same age group, might have led some observers to query why the illegitimacy figures were so low but this line of inquiry did not seem to occur to the commission. To postulate a link between social conditions and social problems, not to mention personal behaviour, would have been ideologically impossible for a clergy and middle class infused with the ethos of Victorian morality. The lack of concern on the part of the hierarchy for the plight of the poor is explicable in the context of a clerical near-monopoly of welfare services, such as they were, through the network of charitable organisations. These organisations were not only inadequate but also punitive and repressive. To stress, or even allude to, the desperate plight of the poor would not only expose the minimal nature of church provision but raise the spectre of state intervention. This is a far cry from current church policy, as expressed in successive budget submissions, which argues for greater state intervention. The 1931 Carrigan Report was an admission that the clergy were unable to control their flock in the all-important area of sexual morality and that the state would have to take punitive measures before things got out of hand.

The only factual evidence produced in the report to support the demand for more repressive legislation related to the claim that the level of illegitimate births had risen sharply since the foundation of the Free State. Figures based upon total annual births showed a 29% increase between 1912 and 1927. But as total annual births show considerable variation (emigration being an important factor in the Irish case) the figures were not comparable from year to year. It is now accepted that the most accurate method is to measure birth rate per 1,000 among single and widowed women who are the actual population concerned. This shows an ambiguous picture of a fluctuating rate, only slightly higher in 1927 than in 1872. But figures on illegitimacy are notoriously difficult to interpret in terms of their sociological significance. It is clear that in times of war figures tend to rise, but no conclusions can be drawn on the relationship between these figures and levels of morality since the latter notion is entirely subjective. What does stand out in the Irish case, however, is the clear relationship between the level of emigration and the figures on illegitimacy. As emigration falls – as it did between 1926 and 1933 – the level of illegitimate births rises. The lowest level reached after independence was in the fifties when emigration was at its highest since the Famine.

Copies of the Carrigan Report were printed up in the normal way, but it was decided that the contents could prove embarrassing if made public. Department of Justice officials were dismissive of it; as one official memorandum put it:

> Unless these statements are exaggerated (as they might easily have been owing to the anxiety of the reverend gentlemen to present a strong case to the committee), the obvious conclusion to be drawn is that the ordinary feelings

of decency and the influence of religion have failed in this country and that
the only remedy is by way of police action. It is clearly undesirable that such
a view of conditions in the Saorstát should be given wide circulation.

The civil servants were particularly scathing of the attempt to link immorality with
the existence of unlicensed dance halls: This section of the report wanders some
way from the terms of reference. The committee might equally have concerned
itself with housing, education, unemployment or any other matter which might
have had an indirect effect on prostitution and immorality. Their suggestions
amount almost to a suppression of public dancing. In its conclusion, the memo
comes out firmly against increased repression as a means of enforcing morality:
'On the whole the report should be taken with reserve: their recommendations are
invariably to increase penalties, create offences, and remove existing safeguards
for people charged: their main concern seems to be to secure convictions'.

Action on the report was slow. It had been submitted in August 1931 and
the Departmental memorandum is dated October 1932, indicating that the
Cosgrave government, which had previously shown some courage in the
face of episcopal pressure, was not prepared to move swiftly on the matter,
particularly as a general election was due the following year. The election was
won by Fianna Fáil and the new government, headed by Éamon de Valera, was
soon to show itself to be more than pliant when faced with the demands of
the bishops. The new Minister for Justice, James Geogheghan, agreed with his
officials that the report should not be published and expressed serious doubts as
to the picture of the country it presented when he submitted it to the Executive
Council (the cabinet). Instead of immediate action, an all-party committee was
set up to make recommendations. The committee met in secret; its membership
was never revealed, nor were its recommendations. The senate went to great
lengths when the Criminal Law Amendment Bill was being debated some two
years later to avoid discussing the report or the conclusions of the all-party
committee. Indeed, when reading the senate record, it is often difficult to
identify the subject being discussed so dense are the circumlocutions.

In December 1932 Geogheghan met with the bishops who put their case for
legislation as proposed in the report. The problems discussed embraced the
usual litany of clerical obsessions: dance halls, the age of consent, prostitution,
motor cars and immoral behaviour on the public highway. The government
obviously took the 'motor car scandal' seriously but faced insurmountable
difficulties in drafting legislation. Not only was car ownership a middle-class
privilege but it was impossible to restrict the use of cars or even legislate for the
behaviour of individuals within a vehicle. The ingenious solution was to define
a motor car as a street in the paragraph dealing with soliciting and importuning

in the bill: 'The word street in this section (shall) include a motor car, carriage or other vehicle'. This allowed the police to treat a car as a public place and use their discretion as to the nature of behaviour within. The Alice-in-Wonderland nature of this logic led one senator to suggest, with tongue in cheek, that a wheelbarrow was a street and therefore could be used for an immoral purpose.

Meanwhile the pressure for constraints on the dance halls was becoming intense. The Gaelic League re-launched its anti-jazz campaign in 1934 with a statement very much in tune with the sentiments of the bishops:

> It is this music and verse that the Gaelic League is determined to crush …its influence is denationalising in that its references are to things foreign to Irishmen: that it is the present-day instrument of social degradations all too plain, even in Ireland. That was the reason for their launching of the anti-jazz campaign, the reason it received the blessing of the church and the approval of the state.

The League was quick to condemn politicians who were seen as behaving in an 'anti-national' fashion. The Secretary of the League, attacking the broadcasting of jazz on Irish radio, had this to say about the minister responsible: 'Our Minister of Finance has a soul buried in jazz and is selling the musical soul of the nation for the dividends of sponsored jazz programmes. He is jazzing every night of the week'. A number of county councils adopted resolutions condemning jazz and all-night dancing and District Justices took up the refrain talking of the dangers of 'nigger music' and the orgy of unrestricted all-night dances. In January 1934 a large demonstration took place in Mohill, County Leitrim. It was made up mostly of young people and the press estimated the attendance at 3,000, with five bands and banners inscribed with 'Down with jazz' and 'Out with paganism'. Support came from church and state. A letter from Cardinal MacRory was read out:

> I heartily wish success to the Co. Leitrim executive of the Gaelic League in its campaign against all-night jazz dancing. I know nothing about jazz dancing except that I understand that they are suggestive and demoralising: but jazz apart, all night dances are objectionable on many grounds and in country districts and small towns are a fruitful source of scandal and ruin, spiritual and temporal. To how many poor innocent young girls have they not been an occasion of irreparable disgrace and lifelong sorrow?

The campaign was given official state blessing in a letter from De Valera, who wrote that 'I sincerely hope that the efforts of Conradh na Gaeilge in your county to restore national forms of dancing will be successful, and within the reasonable hours which have always been associated with Irish entertainment.

It was eventually decided that dance halls should be the subject of separate legislation, which was passed in 1935 without debate in the Dáil. The act was draconian, making it practically impossible to hold dances without the sanction of the trinity of clergy, police and judiciary. With its passing, the hierarchy could rest content that its proposals for the legal control of personal morality had, without serious modification, been transformed into law. But like many laws in Ireland it was probably honoured more in the breach than in the observance. Enforcement seems to have been patchy and the overall effect is hard to assess.

Chapter Twelve

Internal tamponage, hockey parturition and mixed athletics

Margaret Ó hÓgartaigh

In 1934 the National Athletic and Cycling Association (NACA) suggested hosting a women's 100 yards sprint as part of their national championships. The response to this innovation reveals a lot about the position of women in Irish society at that time. Discussion frequently centred on the attire to be worn by sportswomen. Given the restrictions on women's movements, it is easy to underestimate the sporting spaces that women could inhabit.

Athletics for women had been introduced at the Olympic Games in 1928 after the retirement of the founder of the modern Olympic movement, Baron Pierre de Courbetin, who had very clear views on the place of women in sport. He declared that 'women have but one task, that of the role of crowning the winner with garlands, as was their role in ancient Greece'. By 1956, the longest women's race on the programme was 220 yards (200 metres). The 3,000 metres and marathon were only introduced in 1984. The 3,000 metres steeplechase will be introduced in 2008.

In Ireland, leading the fray against mixed athletics in 1934 was Revd John Charles McQuaid, then president of Blackrock College, a Catholic boys' school run by the Holy Ghost Fathers. In a letter to the *Irish Press* on 24 February 1934, which was also published in *The Irish Times* the same day, he made it clear that 'the issue is not: in what forms of athletic sport may women or girls indulge, with safety to their well-being. That question should be duly determined by medical science, rightly so called'. Neither, he argued, was it a question of female activity within their own colleges and associations; that 'question should be duly solved by the principles both of Christian modesty and of true medical science'. He asserted that 'mixed athletics and all cognate immodesties are abuses that right-minded people reprobate, wherever and whenever they exist'. To clinch his argument, McQuaid declared: 'God is not modern; nor is his Law'. Women competing in the same sporting arenas with men were 'un-Irish and un-Catholic', and mixed athletics were a 'social abuse'

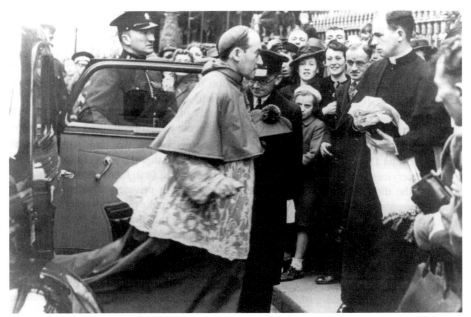

John Charles McQuaid, archbishop of Dublin. In April 1944 he wrote to the Minister for Health 'concerning the use of internal sanitary tampons, in particular, that called Tampax'. (UCC Multitext Project).

and a 'moral abuse'. He then went on to quote the encyclical letter of Pope Pius XI, *Divini Ilius Magistri*, which he helpfully translated: 'in athletic sports and exercises, wherein the Christian modesty of girls must be, in a special way, safeguarded, for it is supremely unbecoming that they flaunt themselves and display themselves before the eyes of all'.

In private correspondence, Father John Roe of St Mary's Christian Brothers school in Dundalk congratulated Dr McQuaid on his 'splendid protest in the recent athletic proposition. Please God your timely action will prevent the carrying out of the monstrous suggestion.' To introduce mixed athletics was an 'unchristian imposition on a Catholic people', according to Revd Dr Conway, the chaplain at St Mary's teacher training college for Catholic females in Belfast.

Writing in the *Irish Press*, J. P. Noonan of St Mary's, Marino, the Christian Brothers teacher training college, congratulated McQuaid and expressed the hope that the protests would 'kill the pagan proposal of the athletic association'. Thus, a newspaper debate was initiated on women's opportunities in sport. The Gaelic Athletic Association (GAA) waded in. Dr Magnier (Cork) supported the views of McQuaid (without naming him), since 'people of influence' asked that women not be allowed to play at Croke Park. Dr Magnier pointed out that from

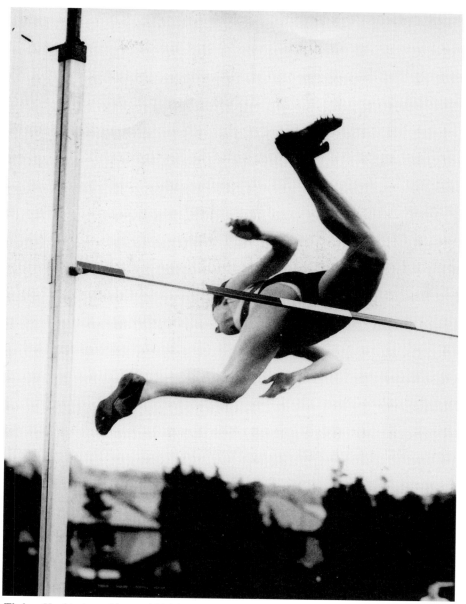

Thelma Hopkins's world-record high jump at the Cherryvale sports grounds, Queen's University, Belfast, in May 1956.

the 'moral point of view it was absolutely wrong to be running young men and women in the same field in the same garb now effected for these events'. Echoing McQuaid, Mr O'Brien of Clare said that the pope, in a recent encyclical, objected

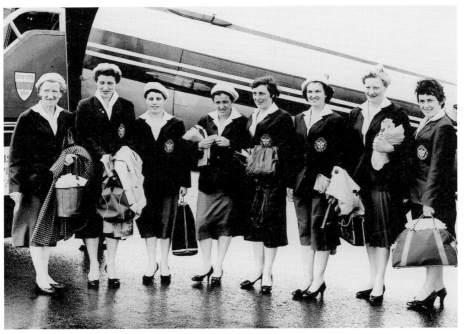

Thelma Hopkins (second left), Maeve Kyle (third right) and Mary Peters (second right) arriving at the 1958 Imperial Games, Cardiff.

to women taking part in tug-o'-war, 'wrestling and boxing competitions but he did not object to them taking part in the lighter forms of athletics, such as running and jumping'. Revealingly, he 'believed that freer mingling of the sexes on the athletic field would do good'. An Ulsterman, Mr O'Reilly, said that in Northern Ireland women had been 'competing in athletic contests for a long time. Public opinion was so much against it, however, that the GAA in Antrim had to prevent women athletes from appearing in Corrigan Park in anything but gym dresses'.

By March 1934, such was the impact of the controversy that the National Athletic and Cycling Association had decided not to implement mixed athletics, although officially they were still in favour of the idea. James McGilton, the honorary secretary of the NACA, assured McQuaid that his letter to them would be discussed at the next meeting. McGilton also massaged McQuaid's ego by suggesting that the headmaster's 'protest was made in the best interests of the Association'. Furthermore, McQuaid wrote to the *Daily Herald* and declared that 'no boy from the college would be permitted to compete at any meeting at which women were to take part'.

The 30-year-old Camogie Association supported McQuaid's proposal. Seán O'Duffy, the organising secretary, reassured the readers of the *Sunday*

Independent that the association 'would do all in its power to ensure that no girl would appear on any sports ground in a costume to which any exception could be taken. If they remained Irish in the ordinary acception [*sic*] of the word they could not go wrong.' Not everyone shared this view, however. Mr McManus thought that 'something should be done to support women in this. They are taking part in different kinds of sport all over the world.' When the NACA decided not to permit mixed athletics, McManus complained about the decision and pointed out that the 'largest clubs in the city have events for ladies—cycling and all'. This seemed to be a minority view, however. The impact of McQuaid's complaints spread to the west. The *East Galway Democrat* explained that 'on the grounds of delicacy and modesty there is grave objection to women taking part in athletics with men, and women should not be blind to this'.

What did the women think? Miss Dockrell, the women's 100 yards swimming champion, thought it was 'hard to understand the ban, since there was no question of "mixed athletics"'. Eileen Bolger was, according to the *Irish Press*, a well-known Irish runner. She did not see what objection could be taken to girls competing in reserved events. A 100 yards championship for girls was held annually at the civil service sports, and an event for girls was included in the Garda sports competition. J. J. McGilton, secretary of the NACA, supported this development. He told an *Irish Press* reporter that, until the 1930s, women had competed in reserved events at men's meetings and no objection was made. The 100 yards championship for women had been in existence for years. After McQuaid's campaign, however, mixed athletics were not countenanced.

A decade later McQuaid, by now archbishop of Dublin, was still concerned about the movements of Irish women. In April 1944 he wrote to Dr Conn Ward, parliamentary secretary to the Minister for Local Government and Public Health, and informed him that at the 'Low Week meetings of the Bishops, I explained very fully the evidence concerning the use of internal sanitary tampons, in particular, that called Tampax. On the medical evidence made available, the bishops very strongly disapproved of the use of these appliances, more particularly in the case of unmarried persons.' 'Unmarried persons' was a euphemism for women. Did men actually use Tampax? Were they seen as a contraceptive device? It requires a remarkable gynaecological imagination to see Tampax as a contraceptive. The more pertinent fear, however, was that women might derive sexual stimulation from Tampax. This reflects the cultural anxieties of the era.

McQuaid's medical advisor was Dr Stafford Johnson, who had studied in Clongowes Wood College and graduated in medicine from UCD in 1914. He took a particular interest in medico–moral issues and was an enthusiastic advocate for Catholic ethics in medicine. Early in 1944, Stafford Johnson wrote to McQuaid requesting the return of the *Catholic Medical Guardian*, which he had earlier lent to McQuaid, 'in which there was given the pronouncement of the English hierarchy on internal tamponage'. With an ill-disguised sinister tone, Stafford Johnson explained that an 'interesting development has occurred. Tampax has been off the market here for over a year and a half. One of our Knight Chemists [Stafford Johnson was a Supreme Knight of Columbanus] has just rung me up to say it is about to be in stock once more but has not been delivered from the agent.' The 'moral dangers' of Tampax were pointed out to the chemist and the crisis was averted. It was 1944 after all! The obsession with female fertility so concerned the archbishop that certain middle-class Catholic girls' schools were discouraged from playing hockey since the twisting movements were alleged to cause 'hockey parturition', that is, infertility. Hence lacrosse was favoured. The latter activity did not necessitate as much midriff movement. While these students were physically active, it was within the confines of an all-female environment. Schools under the management of the Loreto sisters participated in their own sports event from 1905. The Loreto Shield was introduced specifically for athletics, 23 years before women were allowed to compete at the Olympic Games in athletics. Students at various Sr Louis schools played a variety of games from basketball to camogie.

As long as women were not flaunting themselves in front of males, it was possible to pursue sporting activities. The Women's Amateur Athletic Association (a women-only organisation) was to have a particular impact on the development of athletics for women in Northern Ireland. Furthermore, when the Northern Ireland Amateur Athletic Association appointed Franz Stampf as coach in the 1950s, he worked with Thelma Hopkins, who went on to break the world record (in May 1956) as well as to win an Olympic silver medal (the following December) in the high jump. Hopkins remembered that when she first played hockey for Ireland 'we had to wear long black stockings and tunics down to our knees. Really, it was extremely difficult to play. But in the North, we had a lot of support from the men, mainly because Stampfl was there and his athletes were taken seriously.' It may be no accident that Maeve Kyle (née Shankey), who was born in Kilkenny and played hockey for Trinity College and Ireland, did not become involved in athletics until she married an athletics coach, Seán Kyle, and moved to Ballymena, County Antrim. In 1956 she became the first Irish woman to compete in athletics for the Republic of Ireland at the Olympic Games.

As late as the 1960s McQuaid was still concerned with 'unnatural pleasures' associated with female gymnastics, especially the pommel horse. He was apparently unaware of the unnatural pain associated with the event. Both McQuaid's and later commentators' obsession with female activity have blinded many to the varieties of activities in which women could indulge, but the sensual sight of mixed athletics did not become a reality in Ireland until the 1960s.

Chapter Thirteen

'No worse and no better: Irishwomen and backstreet abortions

Clíona Rattigan

Addressing the jury in the course of George J.'s trial for using an instrument with intent to procure the miscarriage of his girlfriend Carrie D. in June 1945, Mr Justice McCarthy told the jurors that for the past ten or twelve years in Dublin 'crimes of passion of the worst character have come before the courts'. The judge seems to have regarded abortion as a crime of passion, which 'reveal[ed] mankind at its worst'. An editorial in the *Irish Times* the previous summer, on 2 August 1944, had also expressed a strong sense of disgust at the number of abortion cases before the courts. The editor reminded its readers that 'Dublin is probably no worse and no better than any other city of its size' and that the city's 'inhabitants are prone to all the many frailties of human kind. Vice lives check by jowl with virtue in our midst, and the mere fact that our people happen to be Irish does not endow them with any monopoly of either good or evil qualities'. While Irish women may have been less inclined to resort to abortion to control their fertility than British women during the first half of the twentieth century, Irish men and women were, as *The Irish Times* suggested, 'prone to all the many frailties of human kind' and a number of abortion cases involving unmarried women came to light between 1925 and 1950.

Abortion was undoubtedly a dangerous procedure at the time; ample proof is to be found in the National Archives of both Ireland and the UK. Some single Irish women became seriously ill following attempts to control their fertility by resorting to abortion. In his deposition Dr Alex Spain, master of the National Maternity Hospital, stated that Ellen T. was 'gravely ill' when she was first admitted to hospital. She was suffering from peritonitis following a 'backstreet' abortion, allegedly performed by Mary Anne Cadden in October 1944. Two cases where investigations were begun shortly before the women died came before the courts in Northern Ireland in 1945 and 1941. Eileen B. made a short statement to police, 'having the fear of death before [her] and being without

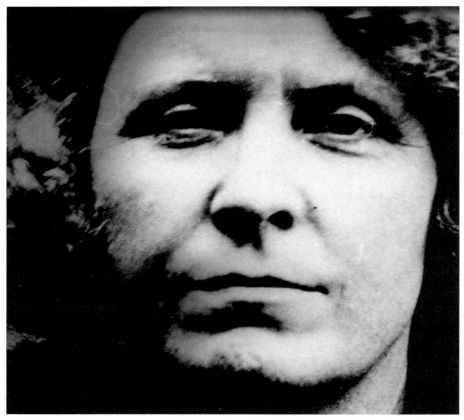

Nurse Mary Anne ('Mamie') Cadden—Ireland's most infamous mid-twentieth-century backstreet abortionist. (National Archives of Ireland).

hope of recovery', and a special court was held at Agnes B.'s bedside before her death. At least seven single women died in Ireland between 1925 and 1950 as a result either of attempts to self-abort or of backstreet abortions.

What prompted them to run such a risk? Single women who sought backstreet abortions were usually desperate to avoid the stigma associated with single motherhood. As reported in *The Irish Times* in June 1944, Karmel M. 'begged' medical student John S. 'to remove the dead foetus because she was unmarried and did not want to go to hospital'. John S. said that he 'had urged her to go to hospital, but she refused, as she was not married'. Karmel's reluctance to seek medical attention in a maternity hospital is perhaps understandable in view of the attitudes towards unmarried mothers in Ireland at the time. The prospect of lone motherhood would have been extremely stressful for single Irish women, particularly for women whose partners were not supportive or understanding

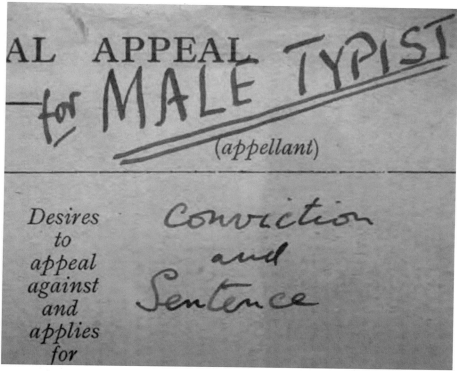

'For male typist', written clearly in red ink across the top of the files of a number of abortion cases heard before the Court of Criminal Appeal between 1925 and 1950. These cases were of a highly sensitive nature. Although much of the evidence concerned women and their bodies, as well as intimate details about their sex lives, the material was considered inappropriate reading for female typists and male typists were employed to type copies of the court transcripts. (National Archives of Ireland).

of their predicament. Judith M. told the court that she had consulted two doctors in order to determine whether she was pregnant. She said that she made an appointment with a second doctor because she felt that she would not get the result from the first doctor quickly enough. She did this 'because [she] was very nervous about it and [she] was rather frightened and [she] wanted to know quickly'. Dennis B. recalled how Karmel M. 'seemed to be in a semi-hysterical condition wanting something done about it' shortly after she realised that she was pregnant. As Mr McGilligan pointed out in court, Karmel M. was 'undoubtedly in distress' when she realised that she was pregnant and began taking ergot, which made her ill. If she carried her pregnancy to term she would have had to leave her job 'without being in a position to earn anything'. Most women would have found it extremely difficult to raise an infant on their own limited means.

Many abortions were carried out by women and often the trial records contain no references to the man who was responsible for a single woman's pregnancy. Between 1925 and 1950, however, men were at the centre of a number of abortion trials. Male involvement varied from case to case. Their input ranged from advising their girlfriends to jump off tables to making arrangements with an abortionist. In some cases, the attitudes and actions of the men with whom they had been involved seemed to have impacted on a woman's decision to seek an abortion. A number of men implicated in abortion cases between 1925 and 1950 established contact with abortionists on behalf of their girlfriends. Men also provided what could be termed moral support by accompanying a woman to an abortionist and bringing her home afterwards.

Access to financial assistance was essential for single women who wished to terminate an unplanned pregnancy. The fees charged by Dublin-based abortionists such as William Coleman, Christopher Williams and Mary Maloney meant that abortions were out of reach for most single, working-class women. Maloney and Williams generally charged between £25 and £35. Alphonsus M. allegedly paid Coleman £60 to terminate his fiancée's pregnancy in March 1944. Financial assistance was vital, given that most women who feature in the trial records worked as shop assistants or domestic servants and would not, therefore, have been able to pay for an abortion or for abortifacient drugs on their own. It is surely significant that four single women who sought abortions in Dublin and Cork between 1939 and 1950 were having affairs with older, married businessmen who were in a position to provide them with money and contacts. Poor single women living in rural areas of Ireland without the knowledge or financial means to seek an abortion and without partners to provide them with money or to contact abortionists on their behalf seem to have been more likely to commit infanticide.

While male involvement seems to have been a key factor in many cases, some women acted alone. Rita N. (21) died in London in October 1925 as the result of peritonitis following an attempt to self-abort. The body of Darrell Figgis, the man responsible for her condition, was found in a gas-filled hotel room just over a week after her death. *The Times* noted that Figgis, the well-known writer, Sinn Féin activist and politician, 'was very upset at the death of the young woman'. He was apparently unaware that Rita had injected glycerine into her womb until after her death. When a doctor who had treated Rita informed Figgis that his deceased girlfriend had used glycerine to cause a miscarriage, he apparently 'looked very astonished, but said nothing and went away very excited'. Rita joined Darrell in London after her attempt to self-abort in September 1925. She had informed him that she was pregnant and that she had experienced violent pains, which she said she could not understand, but she never told him that she had tried to self-abort. She had begun to miscarry by the time she reached London and was later hospitalised. Rita eventually told the doctor who treated her that she 'used a syringe with a long narrow nozzle which [she] got from a chemist's' in Dublin. She said that 'there was glycerine in it and [she] disinfected the syringe before using it'.

In September 1929 Margaret R., 'a pretty domestic' from County Wexford who had been living in London for five years, was found dead. Margaret was four months pregnant at the time of her death. Anne Campbell Pole was charged with manslaughter through abortion and Margaret's fiancé, Frederick J., was considered an accomplice. Although Frederick had been aware that Margaret had wished to terminate her pregnancy (he accompanied her to the residence of an abortionist on at least one occasion), Margaret seems to have made most of the arrangements herself. She had had a successful abortion previously. The judge who tried the case said that while the evidence against Campbell Pole was 'very suspicious' it was not 'definite'. Abortifacient pills were also found in Margaret's bedroom. According to her fiancé, Margaret began taking pills and powders several days before she died. During the trial it was also suggested that Margaret may have given herself a soapy injection before she went to Campbell Pole's house on 10 September 1929.

Unmarried Irish women who attempted to terminate a pregnancy in this period endangered their health and ran the risk of a criminal conviction, while others paid the ultimate price. They were, as Dr Paul Carton suggested in his evidence at an abortion trial in 1931, inclined to 'do anything' to terminate an unplanned pregnancy in a society that condemned unmarried motherhood without qualification. While attitudes towards unmarried mothers would soften over time, abortion itself would, with some very limited medical exceptions, remain illegal in Ireland until 2018.

Chapter Fourteen

'Sisters sentenced to death: Infanticide in independent Ireland

Clíona Rattigan

The County Roscommon district courthouse was crowded in January 1935 when sisters Elizabeth (23) and Rose E. (18) were tried for the murder of the elder sister's infant daughter. Like most of the mothers who stood trial for infanticide in post-independence Ireland, Elizabeth was unmarried. Irish society was deeply intolerant of unmarried mothers and their illegitimate children in the 1930s and the experience of single motherhood was a huge ordeal for many unmarried women. The options available to poor, single women at the time were extremely limited; many felt that they had no choice but to give birth in secret and to take the infant's life shortly after delivery.

The investigation into the disappearance of Elizabeth's baby began over three months prior to their appearance at the district court, in mid-October 1934. The following month, although the neonate's body had still not been located, the sisters were formally charged with murder. Elizabeth E. was one of 183 single women who stood trial for the murder of an illegitimate newborn at the Central Criminal Court between 1922 and 1950; Rose was one of eight women who stood trial for the murder of an unmarried sister's illegitimate infant.

It was not the first time the County Roscommon sisters had fallen foul of the law; in December 1933 they had been convicted of the larceny of three turkeys. On that occasion, they had been discharged. This time, however, they faced the death penalty if convicted. Garda John Salmon was present when Superintendent Twomey arrested and charged Elizabeth and Rose E. with murder in their parents' home. They said nothing in reply. At one point Garda Salmon was alone in the kitchen while the sisters were dressing in the parlour. He recalled how they left the door open while they combed their hair and put their caps on. Garda Salmon took note of the conversation he overheard between them. The sisters seem to have been shocked and confused. Lizzie apparently said 'What did he say we did—murder the child?' Rose responded by saying 'Does he think we are idiots?' Lizzie then repeated the word 'murder', while Rose responded by saying 'Let them murder away'.

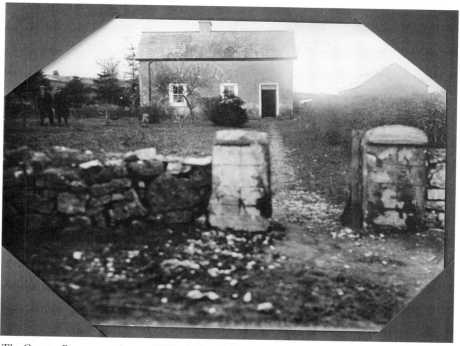

The County Roscommon home of Elizabeth and Rose E. (National Archives of Ireland).

The sisters stood trial at the Central Criminal Court in Dublin in March 1935. After an hour's deliberation the jury returned a verdict of guilty with a strong recommendation to mercy. Nevertheless, less than a month later, on 17 April, both sisters were sentenced to be hanged. Neither sister manifested any emotion when Mr Justice O'Byrne donned the black cap and passed the sentence of death, first on the elder sister and then on Rose. Juries in post-independence Ireland invariably recommended mercy for women convicted of infanticide and judges always strongly supported such recommendations. Between 1922 and 1950 twelve women and one man were convicted of the murder of an illegitimate infant in the southern state. Of the twelve women convicted of murder, nine were the birth mothers. In all cases the death sentence was commuted to penal servitude for life. Elizabeth and Rose would have to wait almost two months, until after the appeal, before learning that they would not be executed. Life imprisonment, however, was an unreality; Rose spent just over two years in prison and was released on licence on 1 December 1936. It is not known how long the elder sister spent in prison.

The County Roscommon case was more complex than most infant murder cases tried between 1922 and 1950. First, despite extensive searches of the

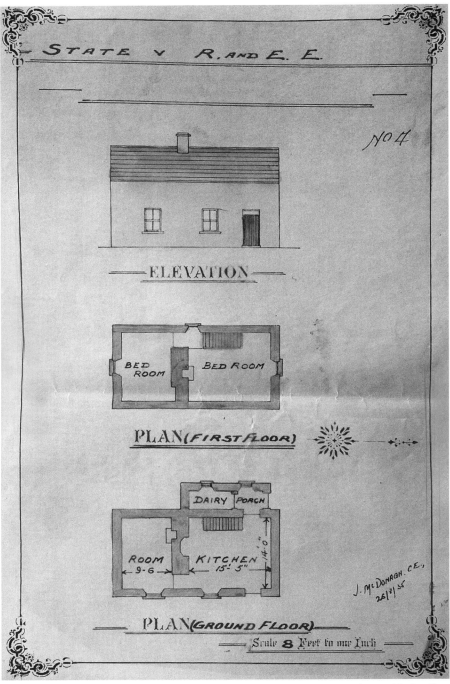

Plan of the home drawn up in the course of the investigation. (National Archives of Ireland).

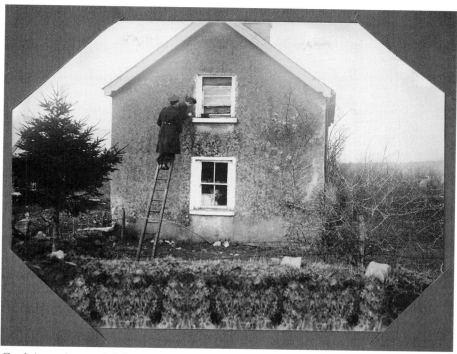

Gardaí carrying out their investigation at the house. Despite extensive searches of the surrounding countryside and the dragging of the river in the vicinity, no trace of the infant's body was ever found. (National Archives of Ireland).

surrounding countryside and the dragging of the river in the vicinity, no trace of the infant's body was ever found. It was not uncommon for investigations to begin before a body was located in post-independence Ireland. Many suspected cases of infanticide were investigated by the Gardaí because of 'information' they received from members of the public. The sexual behaviour of single women, particularly those living in tight-knit rural communities, was closely monitored. The Gardaí pursued rumours about single pregnant women. Members of the neighbourhoods and communities in which unmarried pregnant women lived frequently played a key role in alerting the police about suspected cases of infanticide. It is apparent that while neighbours or acquaintances, on noticing that a single woman was pregnant, did not, in most instances, offer any advice or support, they were quite prepared to alert the police as soon as they suspected that the woman had given birth and no baby had appeared. Nevertheless, unlike the County Roscommon case, the infant's body was almost always discovered before the case went to trial.

Second, neither sister changed her version of events, despite the intense pressure of the trial at the Central Criminal Court, followed by an appeal hearing

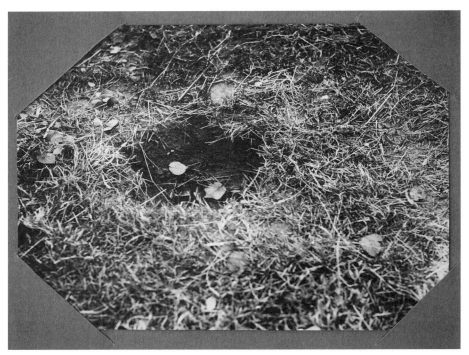

Although Rose claimed to have dug a grave for the infant near their home, the hollow she showed investigating gardaí was empty. (National Archives of Ireland).

and the death sentence being upheld after the appeal. This was most unusual. Women who stood trial for the murder of an infant born outside wedlock often broke down as soon as they were arrested and charged. Few women seem to have made sustained attempts to deny that they had given birth or to lie about their crime; most seem to have broken down soon after being interrogated. Few seem to have thought of convincing lies to tell the authorities in advance of their arrest. This suggests that even if the women who feature in the trial records had planned to kill the infant from the outset they had not considered the consequences of such actions; some simply may have wanted to dispose of the problem, the shame of having a baby outside wedlock, as quickly as possible.

In another case involving two sisters, the birth mother's sister Cáit eventually told Gardaí that her older sister Máire had killed her newborn infant. Both sisters were questioned separately by Gardaí in February 1941. Cáit had probably been interrogated for several hours before she incriminated her sister. When she was asked *'Cé agaibh a rinne é?'* (Which of you did it?), according to Garda Michael Ó Riada *'Dúirt sí Máire'* (She said Máire). *'Thachtaigh sí é lena lámha ar a muinéal'* (She choked it with her hands on its neck). Unlike Cáit ní C., however, Rose

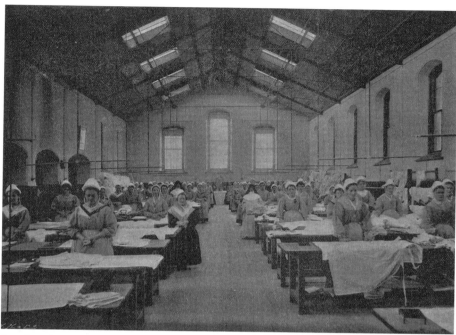

Interior of a Dublin Magdalen laundry in the 1890s. In post-independence Ireland, single mothers would continue to appear before the courts on murder of infant charges, providing a steady stream of 'sinners' to Ireland's network of Magdalen laundries. (British Library)

E. did not yield to such pressure, remaining loyal to her sister throughout the investigation and during the trial. In fact, Rose displayed considerable spirit and defiance when questioned. When asked how she buried her sister's baby, Rose retorted, 'Well it wasn't with my face. It was with a spade'. She never revealed where she had buried the baby, despite having been put under considerable pressure by the authorities.

The sisters also seem to have been aware of their rights at a time when most of the women who appear in the trial records seem to have been ignorant of their rights during the pre-trial process. Very few would have had access to legal counsel during questioning. Yet when Sergeant Tobin began to look around the E. home on 30 October Lizzie reminded him that he was not entitled to search the house without a warrant. The following day Lizzie refused to sign a statement. She said that she would not sign it as she didn't know what she was saying; she was, she claimed, nearly 'gone in the head'. Gardaí had been searching their home and the surrounding areas for several days at that stage.

The sisters' explanations for the death and disappearance of Elizabeth's baby were dismissed by one judge as 'a tissue of falsehoods'. Certain facts have been established, however. Shortly before Elizabeth gave birth the sisters informed their parents and brother that Elizabeth was not in good health and needed to be hospitalised. At approximately 11pm on the night of 2 October 1934 the sisters called to the home of a local doctor, who drove them to the Roscommon County Home, where Elizabeth gave birth to a baby girl, Mary Teresa. Elizabeth wore a wedding ring when she was first admitted and told staff that her name was Mrs M. It was only when one of the nurses remarked that she did not know any Mrs M. in the area that Elizabeth admitted that she was unmarried. Such was the sense of disgrace associated with unmarried motherhood in Ireland during this period that when unmarried expectant women entered the union workhouse or a county home they generally lied about their marital status and registered as married women. Perhaps they may have hoped that by giving a false name they would escape detection after being discharged.

Approximately two weeks later, Elizabeth returned to her parents' cottage by car, accompanied by Rose. Elizabeth claimed that when she got out of the car she put her coat around her infant daughter and left her in a small grove of trees before entering her parents' home. She did this because her mother was in the house at the time. Although the sisters insisted that they brought the baby upstairs to the bedroom they shared ten or fifteen minutes later and that the infant died the following morning, it seems likely that the baby was never brought into the house. In court, Elizabeth asserted that her infant daughter had been delicate from birth. She claimed that the morning after allegedly returning to her parents' home she 'lifted up the child' but 'could find no breathing in it'. She said that she 'cried [her] fill and held it in [her] arms'. Elizabeth then asked her sister Rose to bury the baby's body. Although Rose claimed to have dug a grave for the infant near their home, the hollow she showed investigating Gardaí was empty. She was unable to account for the fact that the baby's body was no longer there.

While some single expectant women, like Elizabeth E., found allies in a relative, others feared how family members would react. Most defendants felt unable to confide in anyone. They did their best to conceal signs of pregnancy from everyone they knew, perhaps even denying the pregnancy to themselves. They usually gave birth unattended. Some women found themselves homeless towards the end of pregnancy; a small number were forced to deliver unassisted in unsanitary conditions outdoors. Many Irish families reacted angrily to the news that an unmarried female relative was pregnant. A considerable number of single women in the case files seem to have come under sustained pressure from their relatives to kill their illegitimate infants and to conceal all evidence of their existence from the wider community. Some were turned out of the family home, only being allowed to return if they came back without the baby. Fear of male relatives' discovery of an out-of-wedlock pregnancy seems to have been a motivating factor in many infanticide cases. It may well have been a motivating factor in the Roscommon sisters' case. In October 1934 Rose E. remarked to her sister Elizabeth that 'the old fellow will kill us if he hears about the baby'. Such fears were articulated by a number of women in the cases examined.

The case involving the Roscommon sisters was but one of hundreds of murders of infant and concealment of birth cases involving a single mother that went before the courts in Ireland during the first half of the twentieth century. Unlike most infanticide cases involving single mothers, which received only passing mention in the national press, theirs was a high-profile case that attracted more interest than most. Many Irish people had followed the sensational case of the sisters from their trial at the Central Criminal Court through to the appeal and the overturning of the death sentence. There was a palpable sense of relief when the death sentence was overturned in May 1935. In that month the *Irish Times* suggested that all Ireland 'is lighter in spirit at the news that the two sisters who were condemned to death for the murder of an illegitimate child have been reprieved'. There was a sense of unease that the birth mother and her younger sister could hang while the father of the deceased infant escaped 'scot-free'. Outraged readers, in letters to the *Irish Times*, decried the death penalty, with one correspondent on 20 May noting that 'if our rulers really do hang these two girls it will be a sign that Ireland is sinking in the scale of civilisation'. Although none of the women, or men, convicted of the murder of an illegitimate infant were executed in post-independence Ireland, many more would be convicted of manslaughter or concealment of birth. Most unmarried women convicted of these lesser offences would be sent to convents rather than to prisons. Judges who tried infanticide cases in post-independence Ireland seem to have felt that convents, or the Bethany Home in the case of Protestant women, were the most appropriate places of detention for unmarried women who had sinned by becoming pregnant outside marriage.

Little is known about the fate of single Irish women who were convicted of the murder, manslaughter or concealment of birth of an illegitimate infant following their terms of incarceration. Some women's relationships with their close relatives may have been ruptured following their arrest, trial and imprisonment, and they may not have returned to their parents' home when they were released from prison, while others may have been welcomed back into the family fold. At yet another infanticide trial involving a single mother at the Central Criminal Court in June 1935, the judge referred to the 'awful plague of infanticide which was over-running the country at the present time'. Single mothers would continue to appear before the courts on murder of infant charges for some time to come, providing a steady stream of 'sinners' to Ireland's network of Magdalene laundries.

Chapter Fifteen

'Unrelenting deference'? Official resistance to Catholic moral panic in the mid-twentieth century

Diarmaid Ferriter

The relationship between church and state went to the heart of Irish politics and society for much of the twentieth century and is obviously of central relevance to the history of Irish sexuality. But the hierarchy was not always strident or, on the surface, demanding. What is most striking is the extent to which politicians continually asked for guidance.

When a government committee had investigated the incidence of venereal disease in the Irish Free State in 1927, a meeting was arranged between a government representative and Archbishop Edward Byrne of Dublin, who was 'hesitant in giving an opinion either for or against publication' of the VD report; after pressure from the government representative, however, Byrne 'made it clear he rather favoured postponement of publication'. The government acquiesced. In 1932, in the aftermath of the Carrigan Committee's report, which investigated whether a revision of the law was required regarding sexual offences against young people and in relation to juvenile prostitution, Minister for Justice James Geoghegan instigated a meeting with the bishops to discuss changes in the law and informed them that he wanted a bill 'which would bring the law into accord with the best Catholic practice and teaching on these subjects'.

There are many other examples that could be given of this unofficial, behind-the-scenes deference, but there is also documentation revealing occasions when the church did not get its way and tensions arose around the issue of who was best positioned to police Irish sexual behaviour. What has been overlooked in particular is the private scepticism on the part of some civil servants and politicians in reaction to what they perceived as exaggerated scaremongering about sexual morality.

In a memorandum prepared in the Department of Justice in July 1938 by its secretary, Stephen Roche, in the context of the possible appointment of women police officers, reference was made to a 'rather alarming document' received

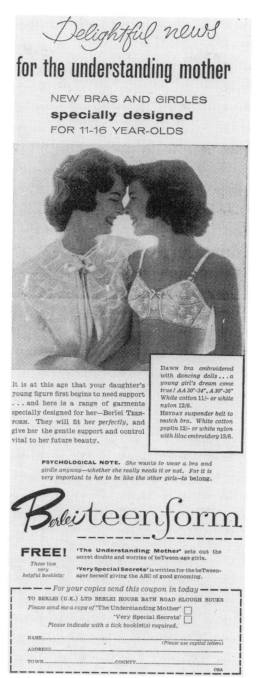

McQuaid was disappointed that the state was not doing more to prevent the circulation of such advertisements. (Observer, 3 April 1960)

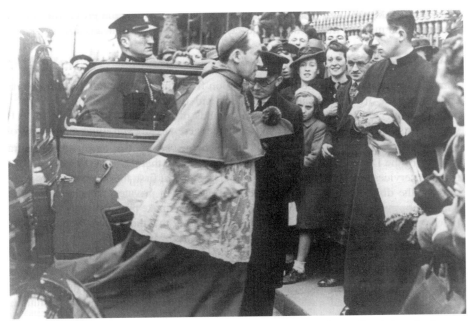

John Charles McQuaid was vocal on matters relating to sexual morality before he became archbishop of Dublin in 1940.

the previous month, which suggested that 'offences against morality were increasing in that city [Cork] to a really serious extent'. Several Catholic priests, Protestant and Presbyterian clergymen and representatives of other social and religious organisations in the city had signed the document. Roche elaborated:

> On the other hand, it was not signed by the Catholic bishop (Dr Cohalan). I learned afterwards that the bishop knew of it and didn't like it. I wrote to the local DJ [district justice], Mr D. B. Sullivan, and his reply confirmed, in strong terms, the suggestion that there was something seriously wrong in Cork and in particular he referred to the number of young girls who had come before him in connection with offences of this class, their apparent shamelessness and their readiness to commit perjury. I then asked Assistant Justice [Henry] McCarthy, in whose ability and discretion I have great confidence, to go down to Cork and investigate matters on the spot (he had just returned from Geneva where he had been representing our government at a women and children protection conference). In sum, he seems to think that both the local justice and the petitioners have exaggerated the gravity of the situation but that there is a lot of immorality and need for some action. Personally, my habit of thought is to be rather sceptical as to the results of state interference in these matters. I have the feeling that the

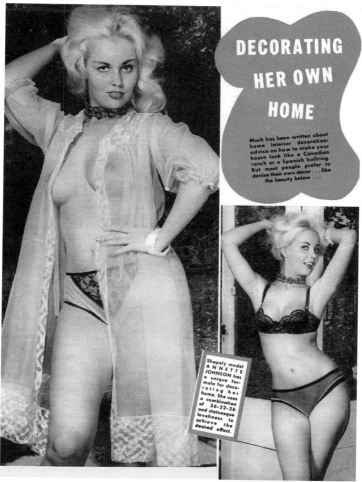

DECORATING HER OWN HOME

Much has been written about home interior decoration: advice on how to make your house look like a Canadian ranch or a Spanish bullring. But most people prefer to devise their own decor . . . like the beauty below . . .

Shapely model ANNETTE JOHNSON has a unique formula for decorating her home. She uses a combination of 36-22-36 and statuesque loveliness to achieve the desired effect.

British glamour model Annette Johnson, who featured in an 8mm home movie, Dream of Annette. In 1965 McQuaid made representations to the Department of Justice objecting to the distribution in Ireland of advertising material for the film. (Parade, 20 February 1965)

rising generation in Cork are going pagan despite all that the churches and the teachers and the voluntary organisations can do; the situation cannot be served by the appointment of a few more state officers, whether men or women. So far as I can see, what the petitioners are really looking for is a body of special police who will patrol the streets of Cork, asking young girls where they are going and sending them home if they are not satisfied with the answers. There is no power in law for any officer to do this and the general theory of the law is that people can be as immoral as they like provided they do not come up against some special provision of the law.

Such frankness was unusual, and he touched upon a number of issues that were relevant to the degree of 'moral panic' that had been highlighted in the government inquiry into venereal diseases and the Carrigan Report. Roche was clearly sceptical about how justified such panics were and how far the law could extend, and was conscious of the need for the state to be mindful of the civil rights of its citizens, a preoccupation of officials in the Department of Justice that had also surfaced in relation to the issue of raids on suspected brothels. There was also an underlying sense of the state wanting to wash its hands of this, on the grounds that if the first line of moral defence—the Catholic Church—could not prevent these activities, how was the state going to deal with them?

Roche was no radical on these issues. In his fawning correspondence with the archbishop of Dublin, John Charles McQuaid, concerning censorship, he suggested regarding their contacts that 'there is no pleasanter privilege attached to my duties . . . do please give me a summons over the telephone anytime you want me to call'. But in truth, Roche and other civil servants were wary of the zealots intent on returning Ireland to a (mythical) state of sexual purity and chastity. There is also evidence that, in relation to pornography and horror comics, civil servants north and south were privately cynical about censorship and the periodic fits of moral panic on both sides of the border. Humorous, affectionate and satirical correspondence between Roche's successor, Thomas Coyne, and A. Lynch Robinson, secretary to the Ministry of Home Affairs in Belfast, in 1954 revealed their true feelings on these matters. They were dismissive of the idea that the state had any role to play in policing morals. Robinson, for example, believed that 'the modern child is beyond any corrupting influence which the adult is capable of devising. However, mine not to reason why', to which Coyne responded that 'there is no spectacle so ridiculous as the British public in one of its periodical fits of morality'.

In the 1950s, Minister for Justice Gerry Boland was also increasingly dismissive of the hysterical tone of those advocating greater censorship. In September 1957 Taoiseach Éamon de Valera received a letter from the Irish League of Decency requesting an interview:

> This letter is written as a despairing cry from a frustrated body of Catholics to clean-up on indecent books, picture-post cards, films etc. . . . we have done almost all we can—we are still storming heaven—within the law to combat the imported press and film evils, but are being thwarted by the very law itself and so find ourselves foiled to remove sources of scandal from public display . . . where are we? Where do we go from here? We must and will carry on the fight . . . Mr De Valera, for our dear Lady's sake at least grant us an interview that we may show you some of the stuff being sold in Catholic Ireland—it's even going the round in the classroom.

The government response was blunt and contemptuous. In a letter from the Department of Justice to the taoiseach's private secretary, Boland wrote that 'the minister is not prepared to receive a deputation from this body. It is apparent from communications received from their secretary over a number of years that the League have very exaggerated notions of what is indecent and any discussions with them could not fail to be embarrassing.'

During his correspondence with Archbishop McQuaid in March 1960, Thomas Coyne referred to the magazines that were being eagerly embraced by young people: 'If there is one thing more than another about this day and age which I personally dislike it is the apotheosis of the so-called teenager and I believe no good can come of it'. But like his predecessor Roche, despite his personal views, Coyne was consistent in informing McQuaid that the state on its own could not provide 'a wholly satisfactory solution'. Enclosed in the correspondence between them in the same year was an advertisement from the Observer newspaper of 3 April 1960, in which a proud mother and her daughter, wearing her new bra, were beaming at each other, under the heading: 'Delightful news for the understanding mother: New bras and girdles specially designed for 11–16-year olds'. McQuaid was disappointed that the state was not doing more to prevent the circulation of such advertisements and was not satisfied with Coyne's insistence that 'if the state is encouraged or even allowed to become an arbiter of morals, it may be tempted to usurp the functions of the church'.

Coyne wrote about the variety of 'unwholesome thrash' now in existence in Ireland, 'which have a demoralising effect not merely on the weak-minded but on the weak-willed as well and are a greater menace because they are retailed at a price which is low enough to give them a relatively wide circulation'. But it was difficult to name and shame because of the 'practical impossibility of specifying all such publications and the risk that those left unspecified might be wrongfully presumed to have ecclesiastical approval'. Coyne maintained that the onus was on the church to 'check the false emphasis on sex . . . the moral flabbiness and the false philosophies that are so much in vogue. This, as I see it, is a task for the priest, not for the policeman'. He then referred to the bra advertisement: 'This is the sort of thing that cannot possibly be suppressed by the state without the state appearing to make itself ridiculous, which the civil authority is always unwilling to do'.

Five years later McQuaid made representations to the Department of Justice about a company called Heritage Films who were advertising 8mm home movies, including one featuring Annette Johnson 'at her dreamiest best' in *Dream of Annette*: 'One of Britain's loveliest nude models in this very artistic movie, incorporating slow motion and excellent lighting effects'. Unusually, McQuaid contacted Coyne at home, asking him whether he could block the entry into

Ireland of this type of material; a chemist had sent it on to McQuaid, pointing out that it had been sent to all chemists selling photographic material. Coyne informed McQuaid that it would be stopped by Customs if they found the film itself but that 'the advertising material is more difficult to detect'. Significantly, there was also a note by Coyne attached to this correspondence for the minister for justice, suggesting that he was no longer a regular correspondent of McQuaid's, probably because he had reiterated on so many occasions that the state's role in censorship was in his view quite limited: 'It is rather curious that his Grace should write to my home. This is my first contact with him in 1965. At one time he used to phone me and write to me about all sorts of problems'. The tone of his note suggests that he was relieved at no longer having to endure McQuaid's tiresome complaints on a regular basis.

Chapter Sixteen

Ask Angela: Reappraising the Irish 'sexual repression' narrative

Paul Ryan

How sexually repressed was Ireland in the 1960s and 1970s? How did it compare to the rest of the Western world? Clues can be found in a source that exists in plain sight: the letters sent to the well-known agony aunt Angela Macnamara.

Macnamara was born in Dublin in 1931 to upper middle-class parents. Her desire to be a journalist and her life as a married mother of four children combined to see her publish a range of articles on the challenges of child-rearing in magazines as diverse as the *Irish Messenger* and the *Farmers' journal*, but it was her column in the *Sunday Press* from 1963 that prompted a series of question-and-answer features to be published, which subsequently developed into a traditional problem-page column that ran until 1980. Macnamara, a devout Catholic, became an arbitrator for those of the faithful who were confused by a society in transition. Caught between a religion that preached self-denial and modesty and a newly emerging society that promised self-fulfilment and sexual exploration, the faithful wrote in their thousands every year, distressed at the moral standards of the dancehall, the revealing nature of 1960s fashion, and the declining role of religion and respect for parental authority in the family home. Although her more sexually explicit letters were initially censored by her editor, the letters provide a valuable insight into the intimate lives of her readership.

The history of the sexuality of Ireland reveals it to be something of an oddity. No history is complete without reference to the range of demographic characteristics that set us apart. In 1966, for example, Ireland had the lowest marriage rate in Europe, yet it had the highest marital fertility rate. The percentage of the population that never married was the highest in the Western world. Repressive legislation governed contraception, homosexuality and the publication and screening of material deemed too explicit by a political and religious establishment fearful that the walls keeping out a British and European

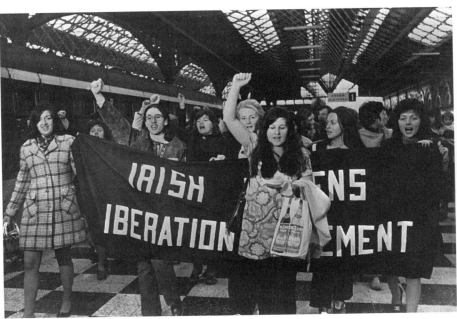

Supporters of the Irish Women's Liberation Movement's 'contraception train' arrive at Dublin's Connolly Station on 22 May 1971. The feminist movement had emboldened women to reject their appraisal at the dancehall and to demand an increased sexual component on dates and in relationships prior to marriage. (Eddie Kelly/Irish Times).

moral contagion would break. The archbishop of Cashel and Emly, Dr Thomas Morris, described Ireland in 1961 as a Christian country surrounded by paganism. The Irish were different. The landmark ethnographic studies of family life by luminaries like the American anthropologists Conrad Arensberg and Solon Kimball confirmed this—that the Irish, in Nancy Scheper Hughes's words, were 'troubled by sexuality'. It appeared that a unique constellation of religious, familial and political influences had determined the sexual character of the nation. The Irish would carry this unflattering legacy for generations, believing that they were more sexually inept, repressed and guilt-ridden than our more sexually enlightened European neighbours.

Much commentary identifies how Ireland 'missed' the sexual revolution of the 1960s. This places Ireland in the category of a late moderniser struggling to catch up, or a country waiting to be transformed by externally led modernising influences. In Britain, for example, a series of legislative measures such as the 1967 abortion act or the decriminalisation of homosexuality in the same year confirmed a nation in the midst of a sexual revolution. Or did it? Despite this legislative reform agenda, how people experienced sexuality at a local, everyday

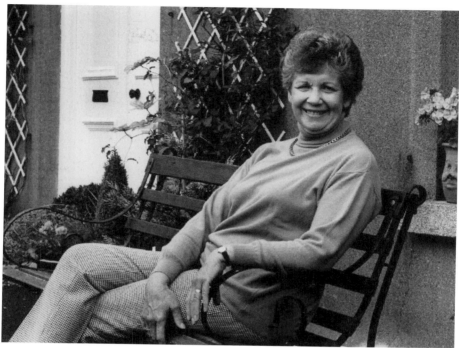

Angela Macnamara, a journalist born in Dublin in 1931 to upper middle-class parents. The letters to her problem-page in the Sunday Press provide a valuable insight into the intimate lives of her readership. (Pat Langan/Irish Times).

level in their communities and family homes told a somewhat different story, one that a diverse range of scholars have sought to explore. Diarmaid Ferriter has questioned the extent to which the sexual revolution had an impact beyond London and the south-east of England, while Jeffrey Weeks has also pointed out that British sexual behaviour had remained remarkably chaste, with births outside marriage rising modestly from 5% in 1955 to 8% in 1967. Surveys of sexual attitudes, like the Latey Committee during the 1960s, also pointed to a high degree of conservatism among British youth, with the majority declaring that they wanted to marry virgins and would marry a girlfriend if she became pregnant. More in-depth research in Britain supports the argument that the experience of married couples struggling to regulate their family size owing to limited access to contraception was not dissimilar to the situation facing Irish couples. One study of Yorkshire mining communities revealed how women were often confronted by a lack of access or willingness on the part of their husbands to use contraception. One woman interviewed, described by the authors as a woman aged beyond her years after multiple miscarriages, told how she had

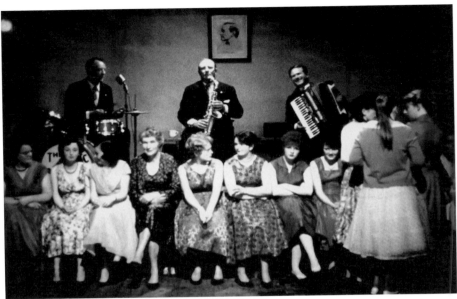

Irish women patiently await the men in a 1950s rural dancehall, as depicted in Pat O'Connor's Ballroom of Romance (1982). By the 1960s women were disconcerting men with a perceived sexual assertiveness in the dancehall and in the bedroom.

bought condoms in the chemist but her husband threw them into the fire, stating that they took 'all the enjoyment out of sex'. Joanna Bourke's study of working-class British communities also revealed a similarity to Irish women in their difficulty in acquiring information about contraception. In the late 1950s the Medical Women's Federation wrote that only four out of 27 medical schools provided undergraduates with lectures on contraception. Letters to Marie Stopes reviewed by Bourke show how sexual abstinence was a key method of family planning exercised by women in the 1960s as the opening of birth control clinics was unevenly distributed throughout the country. The letters reveal that the most common form of family planning after abstinence was abortion, made safer after the passage of the 1967 act. The situation in other European countries was not dissimilar, with France not repealing a ban on contraception until 1967. Mary Evans, in her *Love: An unromantic discussion* (2002) recalled her attempts to check into what she describes as a large international hotel chain in Madrid in 1976 with her boyfriend, only to be quizzed by the receptionist as to their marital status. In the Netherlands, seen as the most sexually liberated of European countries, surveys reveal how sex between heterosexual couples remained traditional, with over 50% of Dutch men reporting an aversion to clitoral stimulation in the mid-1970s.

A review of the letters sent to Angela Macnamara revealed that couples had experienced similar difficulties to those described in Britain. A letter published on 14 December 1975, for example, revealed how abstinence was also used as a family planning strategy: 'Q. I read about "self-control in marriage" recently in your column... we have four children inside these five years and we tried to space them using the safe period also the rhythm, all to no use. The babies still came... I decided there was only one way out for us "Catholic style", to abstain from sexual intercourse. That was twelve years ago.'

While recognising that such a similar plight existed for couples, particularly women, in trying to regulate their families, this is only one story. The analysis of the letters (645 in total) and the interviews revealed alternative stories to the sexual repression narrative. Side by side with stories of couples struggling to communicate their desire for sexual intimacy, held back by inhibition or internalised guilt, were other stories of couples who often also struggled but showed a greater determination to utilise newly available resources to fashion more satisfying sex lives.

For many Irish Catholics who had heeded the message of self-restraint during their courtships, the honeymoon provided the opportunity for sex with a degree of privacy and legitimacy that previously had been denied. The letters to Macnamara reveal the honeymoon to have been an anxious time, with one woman writing on 10 July 1977 that her recently completed pre-marriage course said 'very little about the honeymoon'. Interviews confirmed this; some men shared a similar anxiety but a realisation that their married sex life would be one of learning and sometimes mistakes. The oldest interviewee described little anxiety but thought that 'anything you have to learn has awkward moments and you have to learn the mechanics of whatever it is, whether it is a bike or driving a car, you make mistakes and you have to go on learning'. Another also saw sex as something that could be learned and availed of the wider availability of sex manuals on his honeymoon: 'I remember having a book lying on top of her telling us how to have sex ... on our honeymoon in Paris. That's the truth, it was a learning exercise for us both.'

Macnamara herself, whilst an advocate of sex education, remained suspicious of sex manuals, particularly their use by men. On 28 October 1973 she advised a young man intending to marry and reading a manual that to 'reread these passages for the purpose of making oneself aroused' was not proper conduct for a man on the cusp of marriage. The realisation that sex was a central part of happily married life was increasingly discussed in the 1960s and '70s. Articles, even in the conservative *Sunday Press* newspaper by journalist Gillie Kennealy, warned men particularly that the traditional 'bang-bang' attitude to sex, where every kiss or touch must lead to intercourse, was no longer acceptable to women.

Both men and women were now more prepared to vocalise their sexual needs, to modify their expectations and adjust to the newly communicated wants of the other. One interviewee revealed that his wife rarely achieved orgasm through sexual intercourse and so the focus of their sex lives changed to oral sex, where orgasm for his wife was possible. When I asked him whether this shift towards oral sex was reciprocal he replied 'that he thought it rude to ask'. Not all the men I spoke to were so quick to modify their sex lives: one told me, regarding oral sex, that 'he didn't know it existed ... [it] never crossed our minds'. Letters from both men and women to Macnamara's column also revealed a desire to improve their sex lives. In a letter of 15 February 1976, a married woman in her mid-fifties asked whether it was too late to have a discussion with her husband about why she got so little pleasure from sex. Another woman in a letter of 13 April 1980 speculated whether 'Irish men in this country know how to make love', given her lack of sexual pleasure with her husband. While Macnamara consistently answered such letters in the belief that women hadn't the right emotional context to enjoy sex, it ignored a more fundamental problem that often men, through accident or design, didn't possess the physiological knowledge to pleasure their wives.

Women also disconcerted men with a perceived sexual assertiveness in the dancehall and the bedroom. Letters to the Macnamara column from men revealed that the feminist movement had emboldened women to reject their appraisal at the dancehall and to demand an increased sexual component on dates and in relationships prior to marriage. A man writing on 4 November 1973 thought that there was 'hardly a girl that you would approach who wouldn't go to bed with you', while another published on 11 August 1974 thought that a lot of women 'welcome, desire and encourage sexual experience before marriage'. Macnamara was conscious that the gender regime, so carefully preserved through the segregation of the sexes in schools, churches and social activities, was now out of alignment. She wrote on 4 July 1976 in a reply to a letter lamenting the growing sexual assertiveness of women that 'in all the current talk about women's lib I think we very often forget to consider women's strength and their consequent responsibilities. Once a woman sees herself as a "man hunter" she tends not only to lower her own dignity and the respect of men but also to encourage lowering the standards and sense of responsibility of men.'

The everyday intimate lives of men and women has been the focus of this research. The letters and stories call into question some carefully crafted dichotomies through which we have heretofore understood the sexual history of this period. They question the 'sexual repression' narrative but also the extent to which the 1960s/and 1970s is understood as a period of exaggerated social change. A more balanced appraisal of the period is called for that places Ireland in a wider international context, free from the stereotypes of the past, and that allows for a new sexual history to be written. The research reveals how some couples, rather than being passive recipients of Catholic social teaching, were active in adapting their emotional and sexual lives in the light of new information gleaned from a wider range of media available in Ireland. They were part of a wider debate that contributed to how men and women would increasingly disclose their mutual need for emotional and sexual intimacy. Many couples did enjoy good sexual relationships. And when they were less than satisfactory, some relied on this wider range of sexual discussion, including problem pages, to make them better.

Chapter Seventeen

'Spreading VD all over Connacht': Reproductive rights and wrongs in 1970s Galway

John Cunningham

While the social climate in 1970s urban Ireland was favourable for proponents of contraception, there were obstacles, and activism in the cause might have consequences for the individuals concerned. Galway activists—members more often of feminist-influenced socialist parties than of specifically feminist groups—therefore tended to occupy positions that gave some immunity to social pressure, pressure that was brought to bear by ultra-conservative Catholic groups, prototypical of those that would assume prominence in opposition to the 'liberal agenda' during the 1980s and 1990s.

Galway's population reached 40,000 during the 1970s and continued to grow at the rate of 1,000 a year. Suburban expansion, however, was overshadowed by dereliction in the centre. About 10% of the population studied or worked at the university, which was itself undergoing rapid expansion following the introduction of free second-level and grant-assisted third-level education. Indeed, many University College Galway (UCG, now National University of Ireland Galway) students of the period were the first from their communities to attend university. Within comparable cohorts, dynamic subcultures had emerged – the 'angry young men' of 1950s British theatre; the civil rights activists of 1960s Northern Ireland – and there was a questioning spirit among Galway students in the 1970s. Frustrated by the prevailing mediocrity in the arts, members of UCG's Dramsoc established the Druid Theatre in 1975 and members of its Artsoc established the Galway Arts Festival in 1977 – both facilitated by the availability of adaptable buildings in the derelict centre. Some joined radical political groups, the most dynamic of which was Official Sinn Féin, or campaigned on social issues. One such issue was contraception.

Contraception was legally prohibited, but the Magee case of 1973 established that contraceptives could be imported for personal use, while the pill—available since 1962—might be prescribed as a cycle regulator. On occasion, prior to 1976, contraception made headlines in Galway—as when Labour senator,

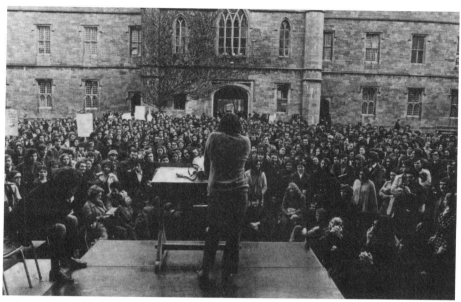

Student general meeting in UCG in 1972. Students, well represented in the ranks of Galway's family planning activists, had some immunity to the social pressure brought to bear by ultra-conservative Catholic groups. (TUSA).

UCG lecturer and future Irish president Michael D. Higgins supported Mary Robinson's 1974 Family Planning Bill (coincidentally, Robinson would also serve as president of Ireland). Higgins' political opponents on Galway Corporation responded by passing a resolution condemning contraception. This prompted the short-lived student-based branch of Irishwomen United to picket the corporation, causing Fine Gael TD Fintan Coogan to react: 'It's disgraceful— women without a ring on their fingers asking for contraceptives to be handed out!' In late 1975/early 1976 the Galway Family Planning Association (GFPA) was established. Chairperson of the ad hoc committee was Michael Conlon, a recent UCG graduate and a supporter of Official Sinn Féin, who had taken an administrative position within the university. Others involved included medical students with a similar political orientation and staff members at UCG.

The GFPA was barely established when the UCG Students' Union (UCGSU) nominated it as the beneficiary of its charitable fund-raising during the annual rag week of February 1976. The sum involved—£1,000—was enough to establish a mooted family planning clinic. Outrage followed. Fifty local residents, headed by Fianna Fáil mayor Mary Byrne, addressed a public letter to the UCGSU: were students' lives to be 'ruled by sensuality without responsibility', and, anyway, could contraception be regarded as a charitable purpose?

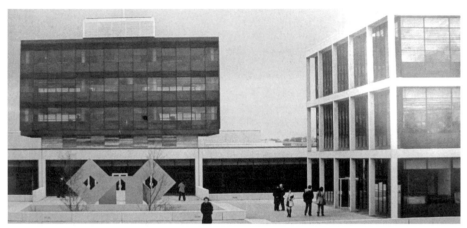

UCG expanded rapidly in the '60s and '70s. About 10 percent of Galway's population studied or worked at the university. (NUI Galway).

All three local papers editorialised against the allocation, with the *Connacht Sentinel* scolding those involved: 'Adolescence and a seat in a university lecture hall do not give people qualifications to determine the case for or against family planning'. In a leader entitled 'Sex and the single student', the *Galway Advertiser* disclosed that student activists had political connections: 'Certain hardliners within the students' union have almost a fixation on what they define as "family planning" in line with the policies of the tiny political groupings to which they belong', an allusion to Official Sinn Féin influence in student politics.

UCG had been a centre of radicalism since the late 1960s, when students attracted by Marxist-Leninism (Maoism) had transferred their allegiance to the republican movement just as it was dividing between 'official' and 'provisional' wings. It was the Marxist- influenced 'Official' Sinn Féin - soon known as 'Stickies' because of their preference for the adhesive Easter lily over the traditional pin-fastened one favoured by their Provisional opponents - that attracted Galway's *soixant-huitards*. Having taken a hand in establishing the UCGSU, they dominated it until 1976, and Galway student leaders went forth to the Union of Students in Ireland (USI) and to the Moscow-aligned International Union of Students (IUS) before taking posts with Irish trade unions. This was the trajectory of several UCG 'Stickies', including Eamon Gilmore (within their party, such veterans of Galway campus politics became known as the 'student princes'). Just before the controversy of 1976, the election of two UCG 'student princes', Eamon Gilmore and Johnny Curran, to the two leading positions in the USI had attracted attention.

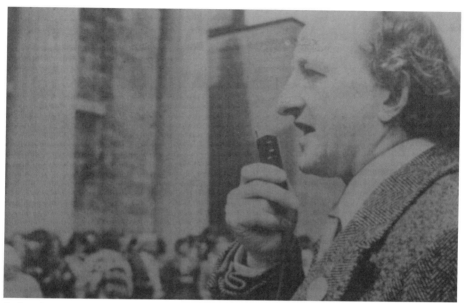

Labour's Michael D. Higgins addressing worshippers outside the Franciscan church in Galway during the 1977 general election campaign. He blamed his subsequent defeat on the circulation of a leaflet targeting him 'by an anti-contraception group'. (Galway Advertiser).

Arriving for work on Monday 16 February 1976, student union president and Official Sinn Féin member Johnny Curran was surprised to find that student nuns and religious brothers were demanding an emergency general meeting of the UCGSU to rescind the assembly vote. In the course of the day, with the support of student Fine Gaelers, the principal campus rivals of Official Sinn Féin, they secured more than the 150 signatures needed to summon the meeting. At lunchtime on Wednesday, accordingly, more than 1,000 students crowded into the UCG concourse to debate resolutions that would have the effect of transferring the rag week allocation to the Samaritans.

Speakers in favour of the allocation argued that a clinic would meet a 'dire social need'; opponents insisted that the earlier assembly vote had been unrepresentative, and that family planning was hardly 'charitable'. Of almost 800 remaining after three and a half hours of debate, 417 voted to give the money to the Samaritans and 379 voted for the status quo. Did the decision result from a spontaneous rebellion by ordinary students or were other forces at work? A front-page headline, 'Opus interruptus', in the student periodical *Unity* suggested Opus Dei involvement, but the claim was not substantiated. Opus Dei certainly had influence—the university was one of its key recruiting arenas (as it was for Official Sinn Féin). According to Paul O'Sullivan, then

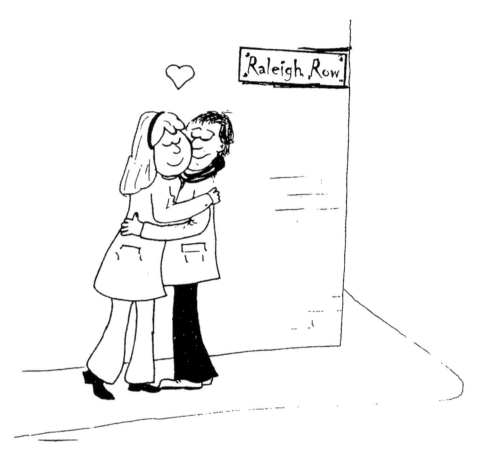

Courting on Raleigh Row – on 21 July 1977 a family planning clinic finally opened in Raleigh Row, offering clinical services and taking over the postal service. (UCGSU handbook, 1979).

treasurer of the UCGSU and also an Official Sinn Féin member, it was Opus Dei that coordinated the political and religious opposition to the allocation, and he recollects negotiating with an Opus Dei representative regarding the wording of the resolution of 18 February. The controversy had an impact a few weeks later, when an emboldened anti-family planning alliance took on Official Sinn Féin in UCGSU elections, and Fine Gael's Mary Carroll took the presidency.

The GFPA's first public event, a 'symposium' in the Ardilaun Hotel on 3 April 1976, attracted about a hundred 'youngish' people, according to the *Galway Advertiser*—men 'sporting fine beards' and 'ladies looking friendly and idealistic'. Announcing that local doctors and nurses were training in family planning, Michael Conlon addressed accusations that the GFPA was composed of 'faceless people'. Because of the 'unfortunate . . . rag week publicity', he explained, they had decided to wait for the 'rumpus to fade' before revealing themselves. There were a small number of opponents of 'artificial' contraception in the room, the most vocal of whom was Deirdre Manifold, a formidable figure and the convenor of a public rosary crusade. These opponents, according to the *Advertiser*, 'were gradually subdued by laughter and, from some quarters, by rudeness'. The rudeness, almost certainly, was provoked by reported threats to 'get at' the promoters of contraception. If it was not evident in the Ardilaun, where opposition came from a marginal group of lay Catholics, the rag week controversy stirred influential opponents of contraception into action. In weekly 'notes' published in local papers, for example, the Catholic Marriage Advisory Council devoted attention to the approved 'natural' or Billings alternative to 'artificial' contraception. Moreover, a Billings clinic opened in Deirdre Manifold's city centre premises before the GFPA was able to launch its own service.

The GFPA's efforts to establish a clinic were hindered by a difficulty in finding premises, owners of the many empty buildings being averse to renting them to such potentially controversial tenants. In one instance an agreement with a landlord was thwarted when an existing tenant, solicitor and prominent republican Caoimhín MacCathmhaoil, announced that he was taking the additional space rather than see it go to the 'politically motivated' leftists of the GFPA, declaring: 'I stand by Humanae Vitae instead of ideas imported from abroad—family planning is based on a philosophy of violence, it is anti-human and linked with abortion'. Frustrated by the lack of progress, three members of the GFPA identified with the libertarian left of the Labour Party took an initiative. UCG lecturers Pete Smith and Evelyn Stevens and engineering student Emmett Farrell decided to establish a stopgap postal service modelled on one operated by Family Planning Services (FPS) in Dublin, using Stevens's and Farrell's Ardilaun Road address. In April 1977 advertisements were placed in any local papers that would accept them offering condoms in exchange for 'donations'. Responding to the claim that hundreds of letters had been received with 'absolutely no negative response', one Michael Heneghan urged Ardilaun Road residents to take action: 'There has already been a letter from the Pope . . . what does FPS need so that they'll get the word, a picket outside their house? But it is curious about Ardilaun Road, why aren't they protesting? It would be interesting to see their reaction if an itinerant family moved into no. 77'.

If Ardilaun Road residents did not respond to the taunts, certain others did. Emmett Farrell recalls being distracted from his studies by Manifold's public rosary group, which convened in his front garden. And there was other pressure. The parents of one publicly identified member of the group, in a village distant from the Galway diocese, were visited by a priest, advised that their son 'was spreading VD all over Connacht' and reminded of their duty to persuade him to change his ways. Michael D. Higgins blamed his electoral failure in 1977 on the circulation of a leaflet targeting him 'by an anti-contraception group', and recalled that, by some subterfuge, the group acquired his canvassing schedule, and sabotaged his campaign by distributing their message in estates and villages shortly before he was due to arrive.

There was encouragement from the extent of demand for the postal service, but there remained the problem of securing clinic premises. A sympathetic solicitor advised that it might be overcome if the GFPA offered substantially more than the prevailing rentals. No sooner had a contract been signed with the owner of a disused leather workshop in Raleigh Row, however, then the man had a change of heart, having received a petition signed by 284 'residents of St Ignatius parish', protesting against 'this so-called clinic'. The GFPA insisted that the contract be honoured and, on 21 July 1977, its clinic opened in Raleigh Row, offering clinical services and taking over the postal service. A hitch caused by the unavailability of the GFPA's original volunteer doctors was overcome when Dr John Waldron, a Tuam-based GP, stepped into the breach.

The GFPA had to transform itself quickly into a service-provider. Steps taken included the appointment of a paid administrator, Dorothea Melvin, and the establishment of a non-profit limited company. An early list of 29 shareholders (thirteen of them women) included seven lecturers/professors, five medical doctors, two nurses, two medical representatives, two teachers, two CIE workers and a trade union official. The majority of the medical professionals were unaffiliated politically; most of the others were identified with left-wing parties—Official SF, Labour and Communist. A significant presence, informants agreed, was that of county coroner Seághan Ua Conchubhair, whose maturity and local stature were invaluable to the GFPA at a potentially difficult period in its development. Opposition persisted, but volunteer nurses Phil Brick and Mary Fahy remember their resolve being strengthened rather than weakened by rosary crusaders outside the clinic. People arriving for consultations also had to cross the prayerful picket line, but reports to early board meetings indicate that a number sufficient to make the clinic viable did so.

Within the GFPA there were differences about the character of the service, with the minority of libertarian new leftists opposing the development of what they saw as an expert-led 'medical model' and arguing for a more emancipatory facility, where volunteer counsellors and medical professionals would facilitate people in making decisions about their fertility and their sexuality. For the majority, however—including both trained medical people and the Official Sinn Féin element—what the public required was an efficiently professional clinical service.

Raleigh Row soon proved inadequate, and larger and more central premises were secured on Merchant's Road, but by the time the service transferred there in October 1979 the context had been changed by health minister Charles Haughey's 'Irish solution'. Thirty years after the controversy of 1976–77, the Galway Family Planning Clinic remains in the centre of Galway, though not in the same building, and the opposition to contraception, though overcome almost three decades ago, is well remembered. Reflecting on the success of the clinic, Jimmy Brick, a family planning activist of 1976–77, drew a contrast with the fate of the other items on the agenda of his fellow leftists of that time. The difference was, he says, that 'Galway people actually wanted contraceptives'. Of the opposition to contraception, he argues that it was counter-productive, because in drawing attention to the location of services it enabled people to avail of them.

The author wishes to acknowledge the assistance of the Galway Family Planning Association, as well as of Jimmy Brick, Phil Brick, Michael Conlon, Johnny Curran, Mary Fahy, Emmett Farrell, Michael D. Higgins, Paul O'Sullivan, Pete Smith and Evelyn Stevens.

Chapter Eighteen

Recollections of the Irish women's liberation movement

Mary Kenny

The feminist organisation of which I was a founding member in 1970 was called the 'Irish Women's Liberation Movement' (IWLM). It is historically inappropriate to call it 'the women's movement' as there were many different 'women's movements', ranging from the Irish Housewives' Association and the Irish Country women's Association to the various feminist Trotskyist and Maoist groups at a different end of the spectrum. When I was actively involved with the IWLM, it was in the full spirit of youthful rebellion against what I saw as a stuffy and archaic social order. Those of us who had been born in the 1940s grew up in a world that was still, in many respects, Victorian. Our parents, aunts and uncles had been born at the beginning of the twentieth century (in my case, my father had been born in 1877, which was before James Joyce!). So we inherited a very traditional social order that was bound to change with the passage of time.

Many of these archaic laws and regulations were by no means confined to Ireland. France, for example, had a 'suppression of contraception' law on the statute books until 1967, and even then it took some years to propel this change through the Assemblée Nationale. But laws were not always observed: people got around them, or sometimes they fell into desuetude. So an over-rigid interpretation of historical conditions isn't always an accurate guide to how people actually lived.

The marriage bar—whereby a married woman was expected, or enjoined, to resign her post once she got married (although it was only implemented in government or semi-state service; it did not extend to the private sector)—had obtained all over Europe until the Second World War. It's important to put the restrictions that prevailed for Irish women into a wider European context. The feminist movements of the 1960s and 1970s (in America, too) were in essence modernisation movements, which were shrugging off older values that obtained almost universally.

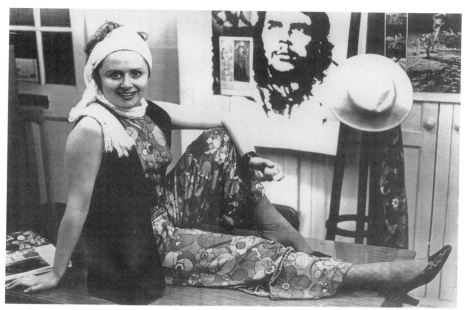

Mary Kenny c. 1970. (Irish Press).

Ireland's time-line was different, mostly because of neutrality during the Second World War; what changed in the late 1940s in some other countries began to shift in Ireland in the 1960s. In Britain, restrictions on married women working in state or semi-state jobs—as teachers, for example—were dissolved during the war, mostly because of the need for female labour. Even so, during the 1950s women in the British civil service did not rise above a certain (often quite menial) level unless they were single. An exception was made for the local postmistress—but in Ireland, too, the postmistress might sometimes be a married woman. The subject of married women returning to work—like equal pay—was opposed by the trade unions everywhere. The male-dominated trade unions feared that the job rates for men would fall if women entered the workforce. There was a fear that the rise of the middle-class woman in the labour force would mean the decline of the working-class male.

Looking back at the IWLM of 1970, the issues that concerned us were several. The more left-wing tendency was focused on housing, which, after all, had sparked the Civil Rights movement in Northern Ireland. Actually, even the bourgeois members were concerned with housing, as we considered it outrageous that a woman could not get a mortgage without the support of a man's signature; indeed, when a young couple sought a mortgage, the woman's income was not 'counted', as it was assumed that she would quit her job when she had a baby.

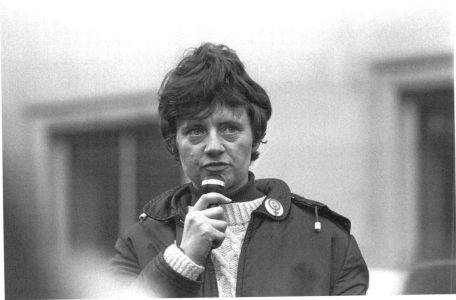

Máirín de Burca—one of the IWLM's most active members—successfully campaigned for the inclusion of women.

This did not fall into the realm of law but into that of business practice. Another business practice that we considered wholly unacceptable was when department stores made credit cards available to women, but only with the countersignature of a man. (This was also the case in other countries: in France a woman could not obtain a chequebook without a male guarantor until 1965.)

What riled us in the IWLM on this question of money was that we thought that women were often more responsible about finance than men, and, as mothers in the home, were more careful about budgeting and housekeeping. Interestingly, the financial prejudice against women was more middle-class than working-class: in working-class households, the 'good husband' quite often handed over his entire wage packet to his wife, and she would give him back his spending money for the week. There have been numerous studies that indicate that middle-class wives at that time knew far less about how much their spouses earned than did working-class women.

The exclusion of women from jury service was a serious issue, especially for one of our most vigorous campaigning members, Máirín de Burca (who was also active in the housing campaign). It was Máirín who provided Mary Robinson with much of the material to get this regulation

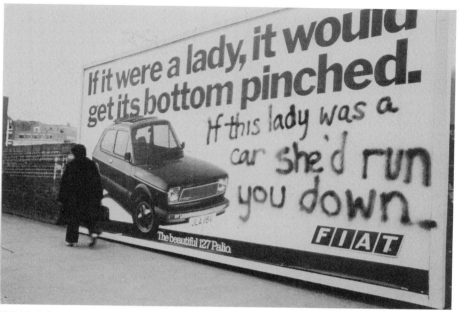

'If this lady was a car…'. Feminist graffiti from 1979. (Jill Posner).

changed. Yet a historical note, again, is appropriate: at the birth of the Free State in 1923, Irishwomen were called for jury service, but so many women asked to be excused that the justice minister, Kevin O'Higgins, decided in 1926 that it would simplify procedures not to call women at all. There was a provision whereby a woman could apply for jury service but, again, it was unusual, and if someone requested to serve on a jury, the defending attorney could object. Nevertheless, I do feel, in retrospect, that we should have blamed our mothers, grandmothers and aunts for not choosing to do their jury duty back in the 1920s and thus causing the exclusion of women later. (On a personal note, I much regret that I have never been called for jury service and, ironically, I am now considered too old: so ageism rather than sexism has thwarted my desire to perform this citizen's duty.)

The issue of getting a barring order against a violent husband was certainly an important one, but a far more frequent problem was the plight of the deserted wife. We thought it a scandal that 1,500 Irishwomen were simply 'deserted' each year—the husband just upping sticks and leaving (often going to England and disappearing into the anonymity of a big city). These women had no entitlements or rights, were in a legal limbo, and had no welfare benefits either. We were also concerned about the plight of the unmarried mother, who was entitled to no benefits (but lots of hostility). Widows, too, complained that they were sidelined and I remember receiving many letters about this. A lobby to support single mothers, Cherish, and an organisation for widows, Cruise, duly appeared and were very constructive.

I do not remember the question of a husband's 'conjugal rights' being an issue. Perhaps discourse about sexual issues was still a little more decorous at that time. It was, of course, considered an obligation of the married state that the spouses be receptive to one another in the sexual arena, but I don't think we were aware that it had the backing of the law. Universally, indeed, rape in marriage was not legally admissible (although any assault is still an assault), but what goes on in the bedroom of any couple can be difficult to police, and the whole point of abrogating the 1935 contraception law was to get the state out of the bedroom, not to involve the state even more in that area.

My own experience of marriage—those among whom I grew up, and those I have known, including my own, over a lifetime—is that, whatever the slogans say, there is no such thing as 'equal marriage'; one partner always has more power than the other, and it is not always the man. I was raised by an aunt and uncle, and my aunt dominated her husband in every single respect—and I imagine that what prevailed in the kitchen, the living room and even the race track (where she chose the horses to back) probably also applied in the bedroom.

I think that caution has to be exercised before making generalisations of power around sex. Men have physical power, but women, in times gone by, often had power of emotional control and power of sexual scarcity, too: many men couldn't get to have sexual relations with women because women controlled what might be called 'the chastity imperative' before marriage. The social and religious prohibition against sex before marriage (strongly upheld by the British agony aunts, for example, until the later 1960s) meant that women had the social power to rebuff males. In some cases, this must have remained after marriage (although individuals always vary).

As single and liberated young women, we all heard married men grumbling that their wives didn't understand them, or that they didn't get enough sex at home, so presumably in these cases they didn't 'force' their wives to have conjugal relations. Pleading sex-starvation at home was a staple of married men out on the hunt for extra-marital relationships.

What's interesting is that we did not, in the IWLM, broach the subject of divorce at all. I think that this may have been (like abortion) a bridge too far at that time. But I think it may also have been that we didn't perceive a very great demand for it. Letters from women readers to the women's pages of the newspapers (many of us worked in journalism) seldom mentioned divorce: money problems, drink problems, desertion and, yes, too-frequent childbearing were the issues to the fore. Besides, I think that the property laws would not have been favourable to women in divorce in the 1970s.

There certainly was an expressed need for contraception, although we have to respect the fact that people had a variety of attitudes to birth control. Over the course of the twentieth century, birth control itself, in many societies, was only gradually accepted. The Church of England did not fully accept contraception, and then only strictly within marriage, until 1958. By the 1940s the Protestant churches had accepted contraception for health reasons, though it also took them some time to accept contraception for pleasure. The biblical injunction to 'go forth and multiply' was widely interpreted by Jews and Christians for centuries as meaning that fertility must be honoured. (Judaism expected the couple to have two children before controlling their fertility.)

By a twist of fate, Queen Elizabeth the Queen Mother played a role in advancing birth control for the Anglican Church. She could only give birth by Caesarean section and after the birth of a second daughter (Princess Margaret, in 1930) was warned by physicians not to have another child. And thus birth control was endorsed for health reasons for the British queen, wife of the head of the Church of England (and that is also why there was no further attempt to have a son).

The historical background to contraception and fertility is part of a context. Ireland's law against importing 'birth control artefacts' was not particularly unusual in 1935 (several American states had similar laws, including the overwhelmingly Lutheran Minnesota). I also suspect, aside from the religious background, that the fear of under-population might have played a subconscious role in hostility to birth control. Farming societies are nearly always pro-natalist: in animal husbandry, barrenness is failure.

By the 1970s, this 1935 law was evidently archaic and needed to be abrogated. The contraceptive pill, which appeared in 1961, probably made a considerable contribution to making birth control laws seem obsolescent. The Vatican had had a long consultative process about the contraceptive pill, from the earlier 1960s until 1968, when Pope Paul VI reiterated the papal view that it was not in accordance with Catholic moral theology (although most of his advisers had counselled him to accept it).

The pill itself was an extraordinary breakthrough in the development of contraception because it was so discreet, aesthetic and reliable. Women could use it without even telling their husbands or boyfriends, so it put women totally in control. And for those (as in the Jewish tradition) who were uncomfortable with the idea of a piece of vulcanised rubber coming between a husband and wife, the pill literally placed no barrier between the couple. Paradoxically, the widespread public discourse about the contraceptive pill was a kind of advertisement for it. And it never fell under any anti-birth control law in Ireland, since, obviously, it hadn't been invented in 1935 and, in any case, it was a medication rather than a 'birth control artefact'.

Some doctors (and perhaps some women) preferred to call it a 'cycle regulator'. For some women with irregular periods, it could regularise their cycles, and there remained considerable interest, among Catholics, in natural family planning (though it was ragged as 'Vatican roulette'). But the contraceptive pill was, clinically, exactly the same product in Ireland as it was elsewhere: clinically, it was labelled an 'anovulant'. That is to say, it suppressed ovulation. The big pharmaceutical corporations (for whom it was a goldmine) were not inclined to label it 'contraceptive' anyway, just in case, unusually, a conception took place and they might be sued for compensation. I think that the contraceptive pill was very widely used in Ireland by 1970, though I'm not sure whether there have been any clinical studies about this. But I remember conversations within our IWLM meetings in which it was suggested that perhaps the pill was too widely used—because there were not sufficient alternatives.

In 1970 I saw these questions as being an important element of going forward and necessary change, and, indeed, many changes were needed and sometimes overdue. With the perspective of history, you see change as part of a historical narrative, which is often more complex than it seems when it is actually happening. Change is a necessary part of life, but there are always consequences to change, and often unforeseen consequences, which will be for another generation to deal with; and here I will just highlight one such example. A woman of my own vintage told me that 'when we got married in the late 1960s, I had to quit my job in the civil service, which I regretted. Yet we were able to acquire a home of our own, in a lovely part of south County Dublin, with a down payment on my husband's salary—I think the house cost about £3,500 at the time. My daughter didn't have to quit her job, but I am not sure if her generation will ever get on the property ladder at all.'

Life is like a Rubik's cube: you fix one problem and another pops up, and fortunate is the person who can get all the squares in line.

Chapter Nineteen

Breaking the silence on abortion: The 1983 referendum campaign

Mary Muldowney

The passing of the 1967 Abortion Act that legalised abortion in the United Kingdom (excluding Northern Ireland) was a source of controversy in the Irish Republic, where access to contraception was illegal. After 1967, increasing numbers of Irish women availed of access to abortion services in Britain while the debate about women's right to control their own fertility carried on against a background of difficult legal cases. In 1981 the Pro-Life Amendment Campaign (PLAC) secured pre-election promises from both Fianna Fáil and Fine Gael to amend the constitution to ensure that abortion could not be introduced either by legislation or by the courts. Many Catholic bishops and priests spoke out in favour of the amendment, but all the other mainstream churches opposed it. Fianna Fáil backed the proposal, Fine Gael was divided, and Labour and the Workers' Party and liberal forces generally opposed it, although all stressed that they were not advocating the legalisation of abortion.

John was involved in campaigning for social change and a more secular and liberal ethos in Ireland. He remembered the political background to the referendum:

> I think the group around—was it the PLAC, Cornelius O'Leary and Julia Vaughan and all of them?—they could see the writing on the wall with the way things were going and I mean the way they did it was actually quite shrewd. They initially got the commitment from Fine Gael and Garret Fitzgerald . . . Fianna Fáil of course had a total[ly] reactionary position on it but they weren't actually intending to jump on the anti-choice bandwagon but when Fine Gael did it, Fianna Fáil panicked and decided okay, we'd better go for it as well.

Many of the activists who were involved in the anti-amendment campaign had previous experience of working to change the laws against contraception and Glenys remembered that their tactics included deliberately flouting the law:

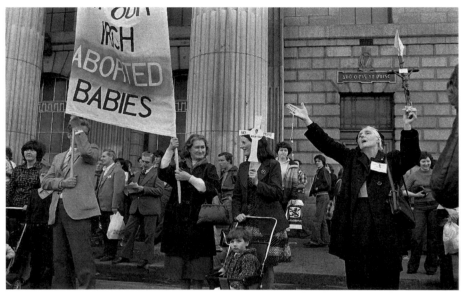

An anti-abortion rally outside the GPO in the early 1980s. (Derek Spiers).

> We got some contraceptives, we got some condoms—and took them to places and sold them. We took them to UCC (University College Cork) and I remember all the security men came and bought them and it really wasn't to sell condoms, it was just to challenge the law. It was just to say this is ridiculous. And we went up to the north side of the city and we had the Special Branch parked watching us so we didn't actually sell them, we gave them away.

The referendum followed nearly a quarter-century of unprecedented change in Ireland but women's rights were not high on the political agenda. There was little evidence of conscious pro-choice activity in Ireland before the referendum, as Alan recalled:

> Prior to that there had been individuals, most notably Noel Browne, the Labour and subsequently the Socialist Labour Party TD, who did on several occasions call for what he described as therapeutic abortion to be available in Ireland but no, essentially it wasn't an issue that was talked about and didn't really figure on anybody's radar until 1980 when a small group formed in Dublin, the Women's Right to Choose Group, with the intention of beginning to break the silence and force the issue into the public domain.

The forces responsible for embedding the anti-abortion position in the Irish constitution were often portrayed as defenders of traditional Irish culture and

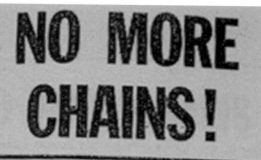

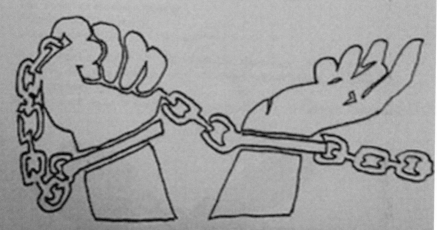

John was involved in the publication of a pamphlet, No more chains! The pamphlet's authors knew that they were likely to lose the referendum, but they thought it provided an opportunity to raise the issue of abortion rights.

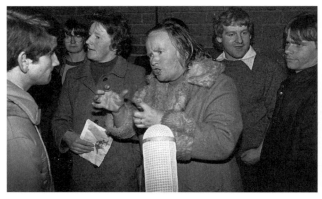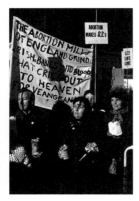

'The abortion mills of England grind Irish babies into blood that cries out to heaven for veangeance [sic]': SPUC banner at an October 1982 counter-picket of a Northside Anti-Amendment Group meeting in the Black Sheep pub, Coolock. The group, which disrupted the meeting, was led by Una Bean Mhic Mhathuna (left) and Mina Bean Uí Chroibín (right), seen here making her point very forcefully. (Derek Spiers).

values. The role played by the Catholic Church and its devotees was an intrinsic element of that defence. Archbishop Kevin MacNamara of Dublin was the author of a pamphlet published as part of PLAC's campaign literature. The following extract illustrates the tone of the document:

> A vote in favour of the amendment (i.e. a 'yes' vote) will be a vote that some unborn children in the future will not be put to death, but allowed to be born and live. A vote against the amendment, or failure to vote at all, will be—whether one intends it or not—to opt for leaving the existing legal protection of the unborn child at risk, and open to an unrelenting and ever-increasing attack.

Anti-abortion campaigners portrayed abortion as inherently evil and there were repeated suggestions that Irish women were being led astray by sinister forces from outside the country. The Life Education and Research Network (LEARN) published a booklet, *Abortion now*, in early 1983. One of the chapters was written by Loretto Brown, a founding member of the Society for the Protection of the Unborn Child (SPUC), and she summarised the perceived threat as follows:

> We must recognise the modus operandi of the anti-life lobby. It can truly be said that capitalism and Marxism are united in the fight for abortion on demand; the one for money, the other for ideological reasons. The average Russian woman has six abortions per lifetime; and in China, women pregnant for the third time are automatically aborted by law. Recalcitrants

are forcibly brought to state abortion clinics while their husbands are imprisoned and the family home locked up . . . We must remember that those who choose to travel to Britain for abortions do so for social reasons. It is inconceivable that a woman whose life was deemed to be endangered would be advised to travel so far in an ill condition.

Glenys had moved to Ireland from England and she remembered that she had only been in Cork for two weeks when she was asked how to procure an abortion: 'It was somebody I'd met and they asked me, I think it was for their daughter, and it was all very hush-hush but the assumption was that because I was English that I must know all about these things and I found that quite shocking too.'

While there was very little possibility of any meeting of minds on the issue, the referendum campaign was particularly marked by the extreme behaviour of some of the pro-amendment activists. Many opponents of the amendment remembered being subjected to vicious verbal abuse on a regular basis but others recalled more violent incidents, including the dowsing of a campaigner with a bucket of what turned out to be pig's blood. Such behaviour resulted in a split between the more extreme elements of the anti-abortion groups and those who claimed to represent the views of the majority of the Irish people.

There were claims by some pro-amendment activists that the anti-amendment campaigners were being funded by foreign forces determined to undermine Ireland's status as the protector of traditional Christian values. Far from this being the case, Andrew remembered how tight the budgets were and the lack of resources available to the activists:

> We used to do interviews, radio interviews and we had to close all the doors in the shop to do interviews because we only had one phone in the building and that was a pay phone and like, that was up the stairs and the bookshop was on the ground floor and we had rigged up an extension to the ground floor so you could use the phone in the shop. But sometimes—it was a push button phone, so you had to press button A . . . Sometimes there'd be somebody upstairs, a customer because this was a telephone for the customers and they'd be on. There was one woman and she used to be on it to chat and you used to get only three minutes so you'd hear "clunk, clunk" as she put the money in. This was the "internationally funded campaign"—and we used to be waiting downstairs for her to get off the phone so we could do the interview!'

In 1983 the focus of the anti-amendment campaign was simply on securing a rejection of the eighth amendment. There was a 53.7% turnout to vote and the amendment was carried by 66.4% to 32.9% of the valid poll. Some individuals and groups tried to raise public consciousness about abortion in the context of women's rights and they felt that the 1983 referendum offered the opportunity to make arguments that might not otherwise be possible. Most of the people who were active in the 1983 anti-amendment campaign believed that there was no need for a referendum to outlaw a procedure that was already illegal. Others believed that the measure was sectarian and were voting against it to maintain the status quo. During this and later campaigns, there seems to have often been a tacit agreement with friends and workmates not to discuss the issue overtly, although there were instances, particularly during the X Case in 1992, when that was not the case. Sometimes there were significant differences with family members that also reflected the experience of activists when canvassing for a pro-choice position. Donal remembered one encounter:

> My father had died a year or two years previously and his sister was a nun . . . We were standing in Daunt Square and I happened to be handing out those anti-amendment leaflets and I was standing under a poster, it was a SPUC poster of a graphic foetus, you know the whole abortion picture. So she came along and a beatific smile came across her. She went 'oooh' as if I'd been sort of rescued from everything she assumed I was. Even though she would have known I was vaguely politically active and long-haired and not quite pious this was beyond her comprehension because when I handed her the leaflet and said "vote no to the amendment" and so on, she completely freaked and her face was contorted into hatred and she said "your father would be ashamed and your father's not cold in his grave" and she ripped up the leaflet and threw it in my face. Now everyone else assumed it was just another mad nun, you know, but it was my aunt . . . and she stormed off. It was genuinely shocking to me—the level of it, you know?

Alan explained that there were differences on the anti-amendment side between those who thought the forces of reaction should be faced down and others who were worried about excessive radicalism alienating the electorate: 'People may not fully grasp it these days, the tension between the cautious and the not so cautious. I was just reminded; during the 1983 referendum the Workers' Party achieved the seemingly impossible. Their leaflet, which was calling for a No vote, not only did it not mention abortion, it didn't even mention women. Now that's caution par excellence.'

The appeal to traditional values that was so successful in 1983 has since been tempered by the understanding that the issue was not as clear-cut as had been claimed. In relation to the X Case in 1992, all the activists believed that the fact that a young girl was at the centre of the controversy was hugely significant because the eighth amendment had been sold on the basis of protecting children and here was a child who was suffering because of that amendment and the state's insistence on upholding it. Rhonda summarised some of the social changes that have occurred since 1983:

> There's been a huge sea change because I think there's been more openness. I mean with the changes, the radical changes that happened—you know accessibility to contraception, you can travel now to have an abortion, and you won't be prosecuted if you're gay, there's an acceptance that society isn't all "mammy, daddy, two children, car, cat, dog and budgie", you know what I mean, that there's not that nuclear family?

For the most part, opponents of the amendment saw themselves as promoting a more open, liberal society in which traditional authority figures would be replaced by political representatives who thought outside the old certainties of nationality and religion. The debate about abortion that still continues is now much more about the practicalities than the principles but the issue is still central to any analysis of women's status in twenty-first century Ireland.

Further reading

Bartlett, Thomas, James Kelly, Jane Ohlmeyer, Brendan Smith (eds.), *The Cambridge history of Ireland* (4 vols, Cambridge, 2018).

Biagini, Eugenio F, and Mary Daly (eds), *The Cambridge social history of Ireland* (Cambridge, 2017)

Bourke, Angela *et al.* (eds), *Field Day anthology of Irish writing*, Vols 4–5 (Cork, 2000).

Brown, Terence, *Ireland: A social and cultural history 1922-79* (London 1985).

Cosgrove, Art, (ed.), *Marriage in Ireland* (Dublin, 1985).

Ferriter, Diarmaid, *Occasions of sin: Sex and society in modern Ireland* (London, 2009).

Inglis, Tom, *Moral Monopoly: The Catholic Church in modern Irish society* (Dublin 1987).

Inglis, Tom, 'Origins and legacies of Irish prudery: Sexuality and social control in modern Ireland', *Éire-Ireland*, 40:3&4 (2005), 9-37.

Luddy, Maria, *Women in Ireland: A documentary history, 1800-1918* (Cork, 1995).

Luddy, Maria, *Prostitution and Irish society, 1800–1940* (Cambridge, 2007).

McAulliffe, Mary, 'Irish histories: Gender, women and sexualities', in Mary McAullife, Katherine O'Donnell and Leanne Lane, (eds.), *Palgrave advances in Irish history* (Basingstoke, 2009), pp 191-221.

Mitchell, Angus, *16 Lives: Roger Casement* (Dublin, 2013).

O'Dowd, Mary, *A history of women in Ireland 1500–1800* (London, 2005).

Ó hÓgartaigh, Margaret, *Quiet revolutionaries: Irish women in education, medicine and sport, 1861-1964* (Dublin, 2011).

O'Sullivan Eoin, and Ian O'Donnell (eds), *Coercive confinement in post-independence Ireland: patients, prisoners and penitents* (Manchester, 2012);

Rattigan, Cliona, *What else could I do? Single mothers and infanticide, Ireland 1900–1950* (Dublin, 2012).

Redmond, Jennifer, Sonja Tiernan, Sandra McEvoy, Mary McAuliiffe (eds), *Sexual politics in modern Ireland* (Sallins, 2015).

Ryan, Paul, *Asking Angela Macnamara: An intimate history of Irish lives* (Dublin, 2011).

Valiulis, Maryann, (ed.), *Gender and power in Irish history* (Dublin, 2008).